# Echocardiography

# Echocardiography

## A Practical Guide for Reporting and Interpretation

## Third edition

**Helen Rimington** BSc, PhD
Consultant Cardiac Physiologist
Guy's and St Thomas' Hospitals, London

**John B. Chambers** MD, FESC, FACC
Professor of Clinical Cardiology
Guy's and St Thomas' Hospitals, London

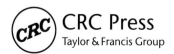

CRC Press
Taylor & Francis Group

CRC Press
Taylor & Francis Group
6000 Broken Sound Parkway NW, Suite 300
Boca Raton, FL 33487-2742

© 2016 by Taylor & Francis Group, LLC
CRC Press is an imprint of Taylor & Francis Group, an Informa business

No claim to original U.S. Government works

Printed on acid-free paper
Version Date: 20150803

International Standard Book Number-13: 978-1-4822-3192-2 (Paperback)

**Visit the Taylor & Francis Web site at**
**http://www.taylorandfrancis.com**

**and the CRC Press Web site at**
**http://www.crcpress.com**

# Contents

# Preface

This book provides a pragmatic approach to clinical echocardiography. It gives a step-by-step guide to performing and reporting a study as an aide-memoire for the experienced echocardiographer or interpreting physician and as a learning tool for the beginner.

Since the second edition, the text has been extensively revised by the inclusion of new international guidelines, grading criteria and normal data. On occasion these are not in agreement and we have then offered a balanced clinical view.

The clinical interpretation of echocardiography has been extended including criteria for surgery in valve disease, and the diagnosis of diastolic heart failure. The integration of echocardiography with other imaging modalities has also been described.

Echocardiography is increasingly used in acute medicine and intensive care units, and a systematic approach to devolved echocardiography has consolidated enough for us to include focused studies in addition to standard echocardiograms. The chapter on checklists in clinical presentations has been extended.

The text has also been reformatted to be more easily accessible, and numerous diagrams have been added. Images and clips have been placed in a web-based archive.

This book will be relevant to all echocardiographers including cardiac physiologists, sonographers, clinical scientists, cardiologists, and clinicians in acute medicine, critical care, and general and emergency medicine. It will also be useful to hospitals and community physicians needing to interpret reports.

# Acknowledgements

We are grateful to colleagues who have provided valuable feedback: Stefanie Bruemmer-Smith, Cathy Head, Ronak Rajani, David Sprigings and Kelly Victor.

# Author biographies

**John Chambers** is Professor of Clinical Cardiology and Consultant Cardiologist at Guy's and St Thomas' Hospitals where he is Head of Noninvasive Cardiology. He has a lifelong interest in teaching and training in echocardiography. He founded and ran the London Echo Course for 10 years, is on the faculty of many national and international teaching courses, and helped set up the British Society of Echocardiography accreditation systems in transthoracic echocardiography. From 1995 to 1998 he was British Society of Echocardiography examiner and he was its President between 2003 and 2005. He was President of the British Heart Valve Society from 2010 to 2013. His research is mainly in the optimal timing of surgery in heart valve disease.

**Helen Rimington** is Consultant Cardiac Physiologist at Guy's and St Thomas' Hospitals. She has long been active within the British Society of Echocardiography, helping to write standards for departmental accreditation and chairing the departmental accreditation committee between 2008 and 2012. She was British Society of Echocardiography Vice President from 2009 to 2011 and helped set up the national quality assurance programme jointly with the British Heart Foundation. She represents the society at the IQIPS standard committees and has been involved in developing the specialist Clinical Scientist training programmes in cardiology. Since 2012 she has represented physiologists at the Academy of Healthcare Science. Her research interests are in quality of life after heart valve surgery.

# Icons and QR codes

A number of new icons and QR codes have been used in this edition of the book to increase its usefulness to practitioners.

 The **ALERT** icon flags up points to be particularly aware of or mistakes to avoid.

 Throughout the book, the **CHECKLIST** icon is used to signal checklist boxes summarising the main information on topics discussed.

 The **THINK** icon marks a point of controversy or where consensus has not been reached.

 A point requiring discussion in an individual patient with integration into the clinical context is indicated by the **DISCUSSION** icon.

The **QR codes** alert you to the free-for-access videos accompanying this book and available online. You can view these through your usual browser using a QR code reader. Some suggested QR code readers are listed here:

iPhone/iPad Qrafter – http://itunes.apple.com/app/grafter-qr-code-reader-generator/id416098700

Android QR Droid – https://market.android.com/details?id=la.droid.qr&hl=en

Blackberry QR Scanner Pro – http://appworld.blackberry.com/webstore/content/13962

Windows/Symbian Upcode – http://upcode5th.en.softonic.com/symbian

You should only download software compatible with your device and operating system. Please note that we do not endorse any of the third-party products listed, and downloading them is at your own risk.

# Abbreviations

| | | | |
|---|---|---|---|
| AF | atrial fibrillation | LAA | left atrial appendage |
| Ao | aorta | LBBB | left bundle branch block |
| AR | aortic regurgitation | LMS | left main stem |
| ARVC/D | arrhythmogenic right ventricular cardiomyopathy/ dysplasia | LV | left ventricle/ventricular |
| | | LVDD | LV diastolic dimension |
| | | LVEDP | LV end-diastolic pressure |
| AS | aortic stenosis | LVEF | LV ejection fraction |
| ASD | atrial septal defect | LVOT | LV outflow tract |
| AV | atrioventricular | LVSD | LV systolic dimension |
| AVSD | atrioventricular septal defect | MOA | mitral orifice area |
| | | MPI | myocardial performance index |
| BSA | body surface area | | |
| CABG | coronary artery bypass graft | MR | mitral regurgitation |
| | | PA | pulmonary artery |
| CMR | cardiac magnetic resonance | PCI | percutaneous coronary intervention |
| CSA | cross-sectional area | PDA | patent ductus arteriosus |
| CT | computerised tomography | | |
| CW | continuous wave | PEEP | positive end-expiratory pressure |
| d$P$/d$t$ | rate of developing pressure | | |
| ECG | electrocardiogram | PET | positron emission tomography |
| ECMO | extracorporeal membrane oxygenation | | |
| | | PFO | patent foramen ovale |
| EF | ejection fraction | PHT | pulmonary hypertension |
| EOA | effective orifice area | PLAX RVOT | parasternal long-axis RV outflow tract |
| EROA | effective regurgitant orifice area | | |
| | | PR | pulmonary regurgitation |
| FDG | fluorodeoxyglucose | PS | pulmonary stenosis |
| HCM | hypertrophic cardiomyopathy | PSAX RVOT | parasternal short-axis right ventricular outflow tract |
| IVC | inferior vena cava | | |
| IVS | interventricular septal thickness | PV | pulmonary vein |
| | | PW | posterior wall |
| LA | left atrium/atrial | RA | right atrium |

| | | | |
|---|---|---|---|
| RF | regurgitant fraction | TOE | transoesophageal echocardiography |
| RV | right ventricle/ventricular | TR | tricuspid regurgitation |
| RWT | relative wall thickness | TTE | transthoracic echocardiography |
| SET | systolic ejection time | | |
| STJ | sinotubular junction | $V_{max}$ | peak velocity |
| SV | stroke volume | VA | venoarterial |
| SVC | superior vena cava | VPC | ventricular premature complex |
| $T_{1/2}$ | pressure half-time | | |
| TAPSE | tricuspid annular plane systolic excursion | VSD | ventricular septal defect |
| | | $VTI_{subaortic}$ | subaortic velocity time integral |
| TAVI | transcatheter aortic valve implantation | | |
| | | $VTI_{aortic}$ | transaortic velocity time integral |
| TDI | tissue Doppler imaging | | |
| TIA | transient ischaemic attack | VV | veno-venous |

# Introduction

## Minimum standard echocardiogram

- A minimum set of views and measurements is necessary for every standard echocardiogram (ECG)[1–4] to:
  - reduce the risk of missing abnormalities
  - help minimise variability between operators and over serial studies
  - provide an instrument for quality control.
- Further views and measurements are dictated by the reason for the request or the findings at the initial study and are discussed in each chapter.
- The template below is needed before a study can be reported as normal. A universal consensus does not exist for the italicised items.

### The minimum standard adult transthoracic study

#### General
- Name and unique identifiers
- ECG for rhythm and ventricular rate

#### Two-dimensional (2D) sections
- Parasternal long-axis
- Parasternal long-axis modified to show the right ventricular (RV) inflow and outflow
- Parasternal short-axis at the following levels:
  - aortic valve
  - mitral leaflet tips
  - papillary muscles
- Apical views:
  - 4-chamber
  - 5-chamber
  - 2-chamber
  - long-axis

- Subcostal views to show the right ventricle, atrial septum and inferior vena cava (IVC)
- Suprasternal view

## 2D or M-mode measurements

- Left ventricular (LV) dimensions from the parasternal long-axis or short-axis view:
  - septal thickness at end diastole
  - cavity size at end diastole
  - posterior wall thickness at end diastole
  - cavity size at end systole
- Aortic root dimension
- Left atrial anteroposterior diameter
- RV size from maximum diameter

## Colour Doppler mapping

- For the pulmonary valve in at least one imaging plane
- For all other valves in at least two imaging planes
- Atrial septum in one plane
- Aortic arch in suprasternal view

## Spectral Doppler

- Pulsed Doppler at the tip of the mitral leaflets in the apical 4-chamber view. Measure peak E and A velocities and E deceleration time
- *Pulsed Doppler in the left ventricular outflow tract. Measure systolic velocity integral*
- Continuous-wave Doppler across the aortic valve in the apical five-chamber view. Measure the peak velocity
- Continuous-wave Doppler across the tricuspid valve if tricuspid regurgitation is seen on colour Doppler. Note peak velocity
- Pulsed or continuous-wave Doppler in the pulmonary artery
- Pulsed tissue Doppler at the mitral annulus
- *Pulsed tissue Doppler at the lateral tricuspid annulus*

# Organisation of a report

A report should include:
- demographic and other data
- measurements (Doppler and M-mode or 2D)

- observations
- conclusion

## Demographic and other data

- Age and gender, heart rate and rhythm are essential.
- Height, weight and BSA are ideal and essential when indexing volumes and EOA.
- Blood pressure is ideal when interpreting load-dependent quantities (e.g. MR, AR or LV ejection fraction) and in patients with LV hypertrophy or other signs potentially seen in long-standing hypertension (e.g. aortic or LA dilatation).
- Include indications for the test.

## Measurements

- Measured intracardiac dimensions are used to:
  - diagnose pathology (e.g. dilated cardiomyopathy)
  - aid quantification of an abnormality (e.g. LV dilatation in chronic aortic regurgitation)
  - determine treatment (e.g. surgery for asymptomatic severe aortic regurgitation if systolic LV diameter >50 mm)
  - monitor disease progression.
- They may need to be interpreted in the light of the size and sex of the patient. Many pragmatic normal ranges are outdated and modern data based on large populations include upper dimensions previously regarded as abnormal (see Chapter 2).

## Observations

- These should be in sufficient detail to allow another echocardiographer to visualise your study.
- All parts of the heart and great vessels should be described. If it was not possible to image a region, this should be stated. This gives the reader the confidence that a systematic study has been undertaken rather than a study focused on only a limited region of interest.
- Preliminary interpretation can be included where it aids understanding (e.g. 'rheumatic mitral valve'). The grade of stenosis or regurgitation can also be included provided the observations used to make the judgement are also included or available in the measurement section.
- No consensus exists about reporting minor abnormalities (e.g. mild mitral annulus calcification), normal variants (e.g. chiari net) or normal findings (e.g. trivial mitral regurgitation). We suggest describing these in the text but omitting them from the conclusion.

## Conclusion

- This should integrate and summarise the measurements and observations to answer the question posed by the requestor. It should identify any abnormality (e.g. mitral regurgitation), its cause (e.g. mitral prolapse) and any secondary effect (e.g. LV dilatation and hyperactivity).

- The conclusion should be understood by a non-echocardiographer and may need to be tailored to the likely knowledge and expectations of the requestor.

- Much clinical advice requires the echocardiographic findings to be integrated with the broader clinical assessment, which is not available to the echocardiographer. However, it may be reasonable to offer implicit management advice in the report depending on the question being asked and the qualifications and experience of the echocardiographer. For example:
  - 'echocardiographically suitable for balloon valvotomy'
  - 'echocardiographically suitable for repair'
  - 'severe mitral regurgitation with LV dilatation at thresholds suitable for surgery'.

- A clinician may need to be informed immediately (Table 1.1).

## Indications for urgent clinical advice

Some findings indicate the need for urgent clinical advice. These are given in Table 1.1.

Table 1.1 Examples of findings at echocardiography requiring urgent clinical advice

| |
|---|
| Critically unwell patient regardless of echocardiographic findings |
| Pericardial effusion: large or with evidence of tamponade |
| Previously undiagnosed severely impaired LV systolic function |
| Aortic dissection |
| Serious complication of an acute coronary syndrome: |
| • Ventricular septal rupture |
| • Papillary muscle rupture |
| • False aneurysm |
| RV dilatation in a patient with suspected pulmonary embolism |
| Critical valve disease |
| Grossly dilated aorta |
| Abnormal mass (e.g. LV thrombus, LA myxoma) |

# Interpretation for the non-echocardiographer

- Findings almost never of clinical importance:
  - mild TR and PR are both normal
  - mild MR with a normal valve appearance and normal LV size and function
  - a subaortic septal bulge is common in the elderly and may cause a murmur
  - trivial pericardial fluid especially localised only around the right atrium (fluid between the pericardial layers is universal)
  - an atrial septal aneurysm or incidental patent foramen ovale in the absence of a relevant clinical history (transient ischaemic attack (TIA) or stroke, peripheral embolism, diving) since these are found in up to 15% of all people.
- In asymptomatic severe valve disease, check that LV size and function is normal:
  - In severe MR, surgery may be indicated for a systolic diameter ≥40 mm or LV ejection fraction ≤60%.
  - In severe AR, surgery may be indicated for a systolic diameter >50 mm or LV ejection fraction ≤50%.
  - Moderate disease may still be significant if the LV is abnormal.
- In suspected heart failure:
  - Diastolic dysfunction does not necessarily imply diastolic heart failure, which is a clinical diagnosis.
  - Estimations of LV ejection fraction are highly operator dependent and small changes should not be over-interpreted.

## References

1. Evangelista A, Flachskampf F, Lancellotti P et al. European Association of Echocardiography recommendations for standardization of performance, digital storage and reporting of echocardiographic studies. *Eur Heart J Vascular Imaging* 2008;9:438–48.
2. Gardin JM, Adams DB, Douglas PS et al. Recommendations for a standardized report for adult transthoracic echocardiography: a report from the American Society of Echocardiography's nomenclature and standards committee and task force for standardized echocardiography report. *J Am Soc Echocardiogr* 2002;15:275–90.
3. Sanfillippo A, Bewick D, Chan K et al. Guidelines for the provision of echocardiography in Canada. *Can J Cardiol* 2005;21:763–80.
4. http://www.bsecho.org/tte-minimum-dataset/ (accessed April 18, 2015).

# Left ventricular dimensions and function

**2**

## LV size and wall thickness

### 1 Cavity dimensions

- Measure at the base of the heart (Figure 2.1).
- A guide to grading LV dilatation is given in Table 2.1.

Table 2.1 Reporting LV diastolic cavity diameter[1]

|  | Normal | Mildly dilated | Moderately dilated | Severely dilated |
|---|---|---|---|---|
| **Women** | | | | |
| LV diastolic diam (mm) | 39–53 | 54–57 | 58–61 | ≥ 62 |
| LV diastolic diam/BSA (mm/m²) | 24–32 | 33–34 | 35–37 | ≥38 |
| **Men** | | | | |
| LV diastolic diam (mm) | 42–59 | 60–63 | 64–68 | ≥69 |
| LV diastolic diam/BSA (mm/m²) | 22–31 | 32–34 | 35–36 | ≥37 |

A recent consensus document[2] suggests that partition values for LV diameters are inappropriate and measurements should simply be reported as 'normal' or 'abnormal'. Individual labs should operate a local policy on how to report LV size.

- If the linear dimension is abnormal or there is relevant pathology (e.g. cardiomyopathy or valve disease), measure volume using 3D or Simpson's method on 2D (Table 2.2).

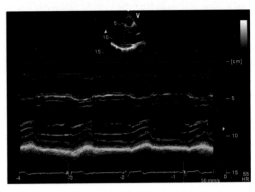

1: IVS in diastole
2: PW in diastole
3: Diameter of LV in diastole
4: Diameter of LV in systole

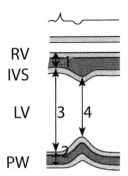

**Figure 2.1 Sites for making 2D or M-mode measurements.** Published normal ranges are calculated using measurements made from leading edge to leading edge. Recent guidelines suggest measuring from inner to inner. Diastolic measurements are timed with the onset of the QRS complex of the electrocardiogram and LV systolic measurements at peak septal deflection when septal motion is normal or at peak posterior wall deflection when septal motion is abnormal.

**Table 2.2** Reporting LV diastolic cavity volume[1]

| | Normal | Mildly dilated | Moderately dilated | Severely dilated |
|---|---|---|---|---|
| **Women** | | | | |
| LV diastolic vol (ml) | 56–104 | 105–117 | 118–130 | ≥131 |
| LV diastolic vol (ml/m²) | 35–75 | 76–86 | 87–96 | ≥97 |
| **Men** | | | | |
| LV diastolic vol (ml) | 67–155 | 156–178 | 179–200 | ≥201 |
| LV diastolic vol (ml/m²) | 35–75 | 76–86 | 87–96 | ≥97 |

A recent consensus document[2] suggests that partition values for LV volumes are inappropriate and measurements should simply be reported as 'normal' or 'abnormal'. Individual labs should operate a local policy on how to report LV size.

# 2 Wall thickness

- Measure at the base of the heart as in the minimum standard study.
- A guide to grading thickness is given in Table 2.3.

Table 2.3 Grading LV septum or posterior wall thickness in mm

| Normal | Borderline* | Mildly thickened | Moderately thickened | Severely thickened |
|---|---|---|---|---|
| **Women** | | | | |
| 6–9 | 10 | 11–12 | 13–15 | ≥16 |
| **Men** | | | | |
| 6–10 | 11 | 12–13 | 14–16 | ≥17 |

*Interpret individually. A thickness of 10 mm in a woman or 11 mm in a man is graded as mildly thickened in guidelines[1] but may be normal, especially in the absence of other clinical or echocardiographic abnormalities

- LV mass is not routinely estimated in clinical practice, but a method is given in Appendix 1 (section A1.1) with a guide to grading (Table A1.1). Patterns of hypertrophy are given in Table 2.4 and Figure 2.2.
- If the LV looks hypertrophied but the measured thickness is normal, this is usually because of concentric remodelling (Table 2.4). This is a precursor to hypertrophy in pressure overload. It is defined by an RWT >0.42.

$$RWT = \frac{(2 \times posterior\ wall\ thickness)}{LV\ diastolic\ diameter\ (LVDD)}$$

Table 2.4 Patterns of hypertrophy

| **Symmetrical** | |
|---|---|
| Concentric | Thick wall and reduced LV cavity size in response to pressure-load (e.g. aortic stenosis, systemic hypertension). RWT >0.42 |
| Eccentric | Occurs to offset the high wall stress resulting from LV dilatation (e.g. in volume-load in aortic or mitral regurgitation). RWT ≤0.42<br>Wall stress = LV pressure × (LVDD/wall thickness) |
| **Asymmetrical** | |
| | Localised, e.g. LV apex or septum |

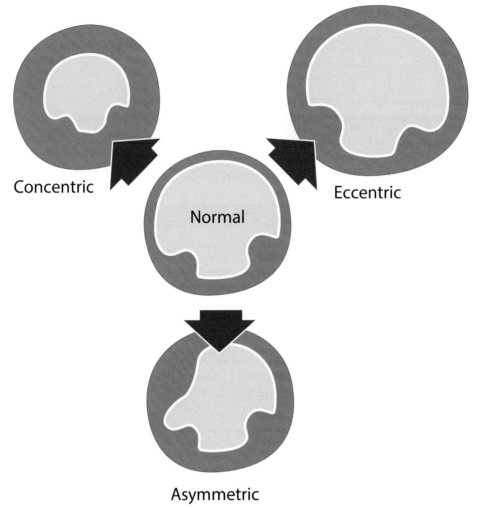

Concentric

Normal

Eccentric

Asymmetric

**Figure 2.2 Patterns of LV hypertrophy.**

## LV systolic function

### 1 Regional wall motion

- Look at each arterial region in every view.
- Describe wall motion abnormalities by segment (Figure 2.3) according to their systolic thickening and phase (Table 2.5).
- Some centres assign a score to these descriptive categories and the most common system is given in Table 2.5.

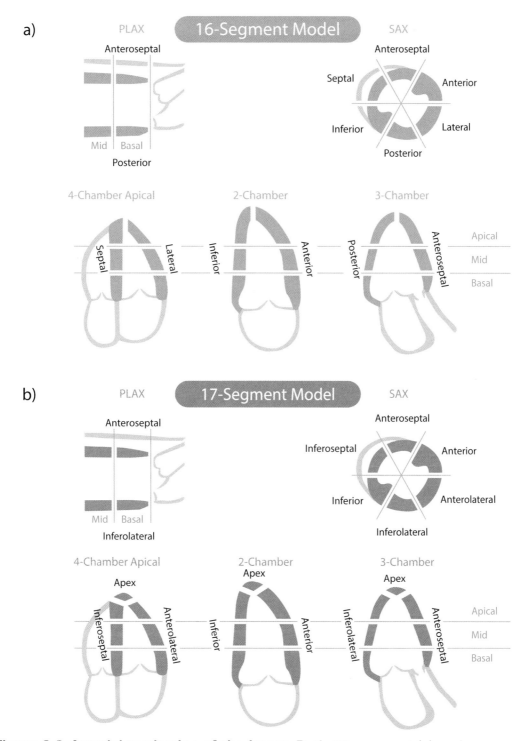

**Figure 2.3 Arterial territories of the heart.** Both 16-segment (a) and 17-segment (b) models are in use. The 17-segment model is particularly useful when comparing echocardiography with other imaging modalities. (Reproduced from Segar DS et al. J Am Coll Cardiol 1992; 19: 1197–202 with permission.)

Table 2.5 Wall motion

| Wall motion | Score |
|---|---|
| Normal | 1 |
| Hypokinesis (<50% normal movement) | 2 |
| Akinesis (absent movement) | 3 |
| Dyskinesis (movement out of phase with the rest of the ventricle) | 4 |
| Aneurysmal (paradoxical motion) | 5 |

## 2 Global function

Some measure of global function should be given. Any or all of the following may be used depending on the preferred practice of your laboratory.

### 2.1 LV cavity volumes and ejection fraction

- With experience, LV ejection fraction (LVEF) can be estimated by eye.[3] A value to the nearest 5% or a range (e.g. 40–50%) should be given since the estimate can never be precise. Quality control against an independent 'gold-standard' is essential if this method is used.
- Systolic and diastolic volumes can be calculated using 3D or the biplane modified Simpson's method (4- and 2-chamber views) using 2D imaging.
- Ejection fraction (EF) is then:

$$EF = 100 \times \frac{(\text{diastolic volume} - \text{systolic volume})}{\text{diastolic volume}}$$

- Contrast enhanced imaging may be needed if endocardial definition is poor and a clinical decision rests on a threshold ejection fraction (e.g. to implant a defibrillator or administer chemotherapy).
- A guide to grading LV systolic function using LVEF is given in Table 2.6 and systolic volume in Table 2.7.

**Table 2.6** Grading LV function by ejection fraction (%)

| Normal* | Borderline* | Mildly abnormal | Moderately abnormal | Severely abnormal |
|---------|-------------|-----------------|---------------------|-------------------|
| >50 | 50–54 | 41–49 | 30–40 | <30 |

*These values are based on the EchoNoRMAL meta-analysis[4] and a recent consensus document.[2] They also harmonise with the diagnosis of isolated diastolic heart failure which usually stipulates a normal LVEF >50%. However, a cut-point of ≥55% for normal has been suggested by consensus.[1] The value needs to be interpreted in individual cases. An EF 50–54% may be normal in an athletic young subject, but it may be abnormal if previously recorded as 60% without changes in loading conditions. The new consensus document[2] gives gender-related ranges for normal (men 52–72% and women 54–74%) and mildly abnormal (men 41–51% and women 41–53%). However, these gender differences are too small to be accurately differentiated in routine practice so we suggest applying the gender non-specific values above and interpreting them carefully within the clinical context.

**Table 2.7** Reporting LV systolic cavity volume[1]

| | Normal | Mildly dilated | Moderately dilated | Severely dilated |
|---|--------|----------------|--------------------|------------------|
| **Women** | | | | |
| LV systolic vol (ml) | 19–49 | 50–59 | 60–69 | ≥70 |
| LV systolic vol (ml/m²) | 12–30 | 31–36 | 37–42 | ≥43 |
| **Men** | | | | |
| LV systolic vol (ml) | 22–58 | 59–70 | 71–82 | ≥83 |
| LV systolic vol (ml/m²) | 12–30 | 31–36 | 37–42 | ≥43 |

A recent consensus document[2] suggests that partition values for LV volumes are inappropriate and measurements should simply be reported as 'normal' or 'abnormal'. Individual labs should operate a local policy on how to report LV size.

## 2.2 Stroke distance

- Stroke distance is measured using pulsed Doppler in the left ventricular outflow tract in the 5-chamber view and is also referred to as the velocity time integral ($VTI_{subaortic}$). Normal ranges in subjects aged approximately 20–80 are given in Table 2.8. In this population the values did not change materially with age.

**Table 2.8** Normal range for stroke distance (VTI_subaortic)[5]

|  | Female(n = 663) | Male(n = 603) |
|---|---|---|
| Stroke distance (cm) | 14.4–28.4 | 13.1–27.5 |

- Stroke volume can be calculated from stroke distance using the LV outflow tract radius (r) (r = LV outflow tract diameter/2):
  - stroke volume = $\pi(r^2) \times \text{VTI}_{subaortic}$
  - cardiac output is stroke volume × heart rate.

## 2.3 Left ventricular dP/dt

- If mitral regurgitation can be recorded on continuous wave, the time between 1.0 and 3.0 m/s on the upslope of the signal allows calculation of the rate of developing pressure (Figure 2.4).
- Normal is >1200 mmHg/s, equivalent to a 25 ms delay between 1.0 and 3.0 m/s (Table 2.9).

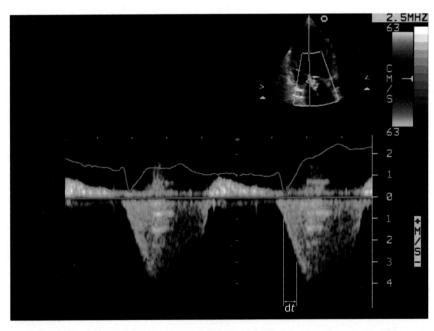

**Figure 2.4 Estimating LV dP/dt.** Measure the time (dt) between 1.0 m/s and 3.0 m/s on the upstroke which represents a pressure change of 32 mmHg [(4 × 3.0²) - (4 × 1.0²)] using the short form of the modified Bernoulli theorem. dP/dt is then 32/dt.

Table 2.9 Guide to grading LV function by mitral regurgitant signal[6, 7]

|  | Normal | Abnormal | Severely abnormal |
|---|---|---|---|
| d$P$/d$t$ (mmHg/s) | >1200 | 800–1200 | <800 |
| Time from 1 to 3 m/s (ms) | >25 | 25–40 | >40 |

## 2.4 Pulsed tissue Doppler imaging

● Peak systolic velocity at the mitral annulus should be assessed at a minimum of one site in the 4-chamber view, but if early signs of systolic dysfunction need to be excluded (e.g. neuromuscular disorder, family screening for inherited cardiomyopathy, chronic aortic regurgitation), then multiple sites from apical views should be sampled (Table 2.10).

Table 2.10 Normal ranges for pulsed tissue Doppler peak systolic velocity[5]

|  | Inferoseptal | Anterolateral | Inferior | Anterior |
|---|---|---|---|---|
| Pulsed TDI peak systolic velocity (cm/s) | 5.6–10.4 | 5.2–12.4 | 5.8–11.4 | 4.5–12.1 |

# LV diastolic function

## 1 What to record

● Place the pulsed sample at the level of the tips of the mitral leaflets in their fully open diastolic position. Measure the E and A peak velocity and the E deceleration time.

● Measure the peak E′ on the tissue Doppler imaging (TDI) signal according to local protocols (e.g. lateral alone, septal or an average of multiple sites).

● Categorise the diastolic filling pattern using the transmitral E and A waves and the Doppler tissue E′ velocity (Table 2.11) (Figure 2.5).

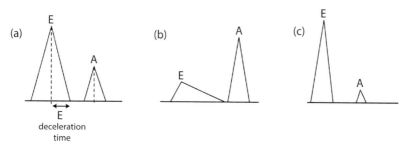

Figure 2.5 Left ventricular filling patterns: (a) normal; (b) slow filling (low peak E velocity, long deceleration time, high peak A velocity); (c) restrictive (high peak E velocity with short E deceleration time and low or absent A wave).

- If in atrial fibrillation (AF), diastole is already abnormal. It is still worth measuring E, E deceleration and E' to look for restrictive filling.

**Table 2.11**     Basic guide to descriptive filling patterns

| LV diastole | E:A ratio* | E dec time (ms)* | E/E' ratio lateral[†] |
|---|---|---|---|
| Normal | 0.8–1.5 | 150–200<br>150–280 (age >65) | ≤10 |
| Slow filling | <0.8 | >200<br>>280 (age >65) | ≤10 |
| Pseudonormal | 0.8–1.5 | 150–200<br>150–280 (age >65) | >10 |
| Restrictive | >2 | <150 | >10 |

*Precise values vary between research studies; these ranges are a composite[8–13]
[†]If tissue Doppler is recorded at the septum,[12, 14] use a ratio of >15; if an average is taken, use a ratio of >13

# 2 Initial interpretation

Interpretation depends on whether LV systolic function is impaired.

## 2.1 LV systolic function is impaired

- The diagnosis of heart failure is made.
- The main concern about diastole is whether there is restrictive filling since this denotes a particularly poor prognosis and might affect the choice of medication.[15] Restrictive filling is sometimes subdivided into reversible (normalises with a fall in preload, e.g. after a valsalva manoeuvre) and irreversible. Irreversible restrictive filling is associated with a particularly high risk of events.
- Further diastolic measures (isovolumic relaxation time (IVRT), pulmonary vein (PV) flow) are unlikely to be clinically useful.

## 2.2 LV systolic function is normal (LVEF >50%)

The description of diastole needs to be extended to determine whether there is diastolic heart failure.

### Appearance on 2D

- Either left ventricular hypertrophy (pages 9, 32) or a large left atrium (in the absence of mitral valve disease) (page 141) suggests that diastolic function is likely to be abnormal.

## Restrictive filling pattern

● Abnormal diastolic filling is established although the cause needs further investigation (e.g. pericardial constriction or diastolic heart failure as a result of hypertension, restrictive cardiomyopathy).

## Normal vs pseudonormal

● Guideline thresholds of the E/E' ratio for diagnosing pseudonormal filling change as data are accumulated. They also depend on the site of recording tissue Doppler velocities and whether a single site or averages over two or more sites are used.

● The likelihood of the filling pattern being pseudonormal rather than normal rises the higher the E/E' ratio (definitely abnormal at any site if >15) and if there is:

  ● LA enlargement
  ● LV hypertrophy
  ● a low peak E' velocity (e.g. <9 cm/s)
  ● raised pulmonary artery (PA) pressure in the absence of lung disease (see page 54)
  ● abnormal pulmonary vein flow.

## Pulmonary vein flow

● Usually, the mitral filling pattern in conjunction with the tissue Doppler measures is sufficient to assess diastole. However, on occasion it might be useful to measure (Figure 2.6):

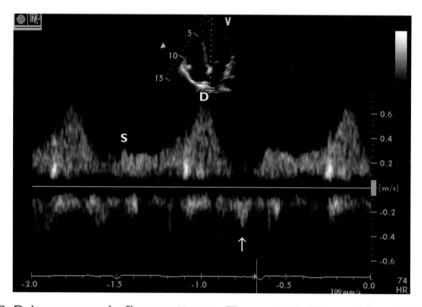

**Figure 2.6 Pulmonary vein flow patterns.** The systolic (S) and diastole (D) peaks of forward flow are marked. Atrial reversal (arrow) has a peak velocity of 0.35 m/s.

17

- the peak velocity of the pulmonary flow reversal
- the duration of atrial flow reversal (PV duration)
- the duration of the transmitral A wave (transmitral duration).
- The most reliable measure of diastolic dysfunction (Table 2.12) is (PV duration–transmitral duration) >30 ms.

Table 2.12 Diastolic function using transmitral and pulmonary vein pulsed Doppler[8-11]

| Diastolic function | Transmitral and TDI pattern | Duration of PV A wave reversal | PV A wave peak velocity (m/s) |
|---|---|---|---|
| Normal | Normal | Normal | <0.35 |
| Mild dysfunction | Slow | Normal | <0.35 |
| Moderate dysfunction | Pseudonormal | Prolonged (>30 ms) | >0.35 |
| Severe dysfunction | Restrictive | Prolonged (>30 ms) | >0.35 |

# Diastolic heart failure

- Diastolic heart failure is a clinical diagnosis for which no firm consensus exists. The core diagnostic features are:
  - symptoms and clinical signs of heart failure
  - absence of other causes of breathlessness including valve disease
  - raised level of B-type natriuretic peptide
  - normal resting LV ejection fraction (currently defined as >50%)
  - suggestive echocardiographic findings, especially LV hypertrophy or a dilated LA.
- A mildly reduced LV ejection fraction insufficient to cause heart failure needs further interpretation and raises the possibility of deterioration on exercise as a result of coronary disease or cardiomyopathy.

# MISTAKES TO AVOID

- Incorporating false LV tendon or RV trabeculation in septal measurement
- Cutting the septum or LV cavity obliquely
- Diagnosing diastolic heart failure from the echocardiographic filling pattern alone
- In a patient with clinical heart failure and normal LVEF, forgetting to consider pericardial constriction. Check for a dilated IVC and septal bounce (Chapter 15)
- Diagnosing systolic dysfunction from a borderline LV ejection fraction in an athletic subject when all other findings are normal

## CHECKLIST FOR REPORTING LEFT VENTRICULAR FUNCTION

1. LV and LA dimensions
2. Global LV systolic function
3. Regional LV systolic function
4. Grade of systolic dysfunction
5. LV filling pattern and E/E' ratio
6. RV function and PA pressure
7. Is there evidence of high filling pressure (e.g. E/E' >15)?

## References

1. Lang RM, Bierig M, Devereux RB et al. Recommendations for chamber quantification. *Eur J Echocardiogr* 2006;7(2):79-108.
2. Lang RM, Badano LP, Mor-Avi V et al. Recommendations for cardiac chamber quantification by echocardiography in adults: an update from the American Society of Echocardiography and the European Association of Cardiovascular Imaging. *J Am Soc Echocardiogr* 2015;28:1-39.
3. Hope MD, de la Pena E, Yang PC, Liang DH, McConnell MV, Rosenthal DN. A visual approach for the accurate determination of echocardiographic left ventricular ejection fraction by medical students. *J Am Soc Echocardiogr* 2003;16(8):824-31.

4. Ethnic-specific normative reference values for echocardiographic left atrial and ventricular mass, and systolic function. The EchoNoRMAL Study. J Am Coll Cardiol Img 2015;8: 656–665.

5. Dalen H, Thorstensen A, Vatten LJ et al. Reference values and distribution of conventional echocardiographic Doppler measures and longitudinal tissue Doppler velocities in a population free from cardiovascular disease. *Circ Cardiovasc Imaging* 2010;3:614–22.

6. Pai RG, Bansal RC, Shah PM. Doppler-derived rate of left ventricular pressure rise. Its correlation with the postoperative left ventricular function in mitral regurgitation. *Circulation* 1990;82:514–20.

7. Nishimura RA, Tajik AJ. Quantitative hemodynamics by Doppler echocardiography: a noninvasive alternative to cardiac catheterization. *Prog Cardiovasc Dis* 1994;36(4):309–42.

8. Rakowski H, Appleton C, Chan KL et al. Canadian consensus recommendations for the measurement and reporting of diastolic dysfunction by echocardiography: from the Investigators of Consensus on Diastolic Dysfunction by Echocardiography. *J Am Soc Echocardiogr* 1996;9(5):736–60.

9. Paulus WJ. How to diagnose diastolic heart failure. European Study Group on Diastolic Heart Failure. *Eur Heart J* 1998;19:990–1003.

10. Redfield MM, Jacobsen SJ, Burnett JC, Jr, Mahoney DW, Bailey KR, Rodeheffer RJ. Burden of systolic and diastolic ventricular dysfunction in the community: appreciating the scope of the heart failure epidemic. *JAMA* 2003;289(2):194–202.

11. Mottram PM, Marwick TH. Assessment of diastolic function: what the general cardiologist needs to know. *Heart* 2005;91(5):681–95.

12. Nagueh SF, Middleton KJ, Kopelen HA, Zoghbi WA, Quinones MA. Doppler tissue imaging: a noninvasive technique for evaluation of left ventricular relaxation and estimation of filling pressures. *J Am Coll Cardiol* 1997;30(6):1527–33.

13. Dokainish H, Zoghbi WA, Lakkis NM et al. Optimal noninvasive assessment of left ventricular filling pressures: a comparison of tissue Doppler echocardiography and B-type natriuretic peptide in patients with pulmonary artery catheters. *Circulation* 2004;109(20):2432–9.

14. Ommen SR, Nishimura RA. A clinical approach to the assessment of left ventricular diastolic function by Doppler echocardiography: update 2003. *Heart* 2003;89 Suppl 3:iii18–iii23.

15. Giannuzzi P, Temporelli PL, Bosimini E et al. Independent and incremental prognostic value of Doppler-derived mitral deceleration time of early filling in both symptomatic and asymptomatic patients with left ventricular dysfunction. *J Am Coll Cardiol* 1996;28(2):383–90.

# Acute coronary syndrome | 3

Echocardiography is indicated:

- to help determine whether a mildly raised troponin level is caused by a new cardiac event or non-cardiac illness
- after myocardial infarction to determine residual LV function and to look for complications
- during pain or with ST segment changes to aid the differentiation between myocardial ischaemia and other causes (e.g. pericarditis or aortic dissection)
- as an emergency in cardiac decompensation to look for acute complications (papillary muscle rupture, ventricular septal rupture or free wall rupture).

## 1 Assess regional LV systolic function

The working diagnosis is confirmed by a regional wall motion abnormality without scarring in an arterial territory.

- Describe the segments affected (see Figure 2.3, page 11).
- Comment on the other regions. Compensatory hyperkinesis is a good prognostic sign. Hypokinesis of a territory other than of the acute infarct suggests multivessel disease and is a poor prognostic sign.
- Are there thin segments, less than 6 mm thick? This implies previous coronary events with non-viable scarring.
- A wall motion abnormality affecting the mid segments and usually the apex suggests Takotsubo cardiomyopathy (Table 3.1)[1, 2] especially in women aged over 50 after an emotional shock (present in 65% of cases).

Table 3.1 Features of Takotsubo cardiomyopathy[1]

| |
|---|
| Transient hypokinesis, akinesis, or dyskinesis of the left ventricular mid segments with or without apical involvement |
| The regional wall motion abnormalities extend beyond a single epicardial vascular distribution |
| Absence of obstructive coronary disease* or angiographic evidence of acute plaque rupture |
| New electrocardiographic abnormalities (either ST-segment elevation and/or T-wave inversion) or modest elevation in cardiac troponin |
| Absence of phaeochromocytoma or myocarditis |

*May rarely coexist with obstructive coronary disease

## 2 Global systolic function

- Report ejection fraction and velocity integral. Both give prognostic information.
- If the ejection fraction appears low by eye, measure systolic and diastolic volumes using 3D or Simpson's method. The systolic volume refines risk and the ejection fraction is used to guide the decision for an implantable defibrillator (usually LV ejection fraction <35%).

## 3 Right ventricle

- Up to 30% of all inferior infarcts are associated with right ventricular infarction and in 10% the RV involvement is haemodynamically significant.
- Estimate pulmonary artery pressure (Chapter 6).

## 4 Describe the mitral valve

- Mitral regurgitation is common after infarction (Table 3.2).
- A restricted posterior leaflet causing a posteriorly directed jet is common after an inferior or posterior infarction (Figure 3.1).
- 'Tenting' of both leaflets leading to a central jet occurs when there is dilatation of the mid and apical parts of the LV cavity (see Figure 8.5, page 83).
- More complex situations can arise with restriction of some parts of the leaflet and prolapse of other parts as a result of stretching or rupture of minor chordae or parts of the papillary muscle.
- Grade the regurgitation (see page 87). If moderate or worse, there is an effect on mortality independent of other factors including LV systolic function.[3] This may affect the decision to offer surgery rather than percutaneous coronary intervention (PCI) after the acute coronary event.

Table 3.2 Causes of mitral regurgitation after myocardial infarction

| |
|---|
| Restricted posterior mitral leaflet (Figure 3.1) |
| Left ventricular dilatation leading to symmetrical 'tenting' of the mitral leaflets |
| Rupture of papillary muscle or major chordae |
| Mitral prolapse as a result of minor chordal dysfunction |
| Coexistent primary mitral valve disease |

## 5 Complications

Possible complications after myocardial infarction are listed in Table 3.3.

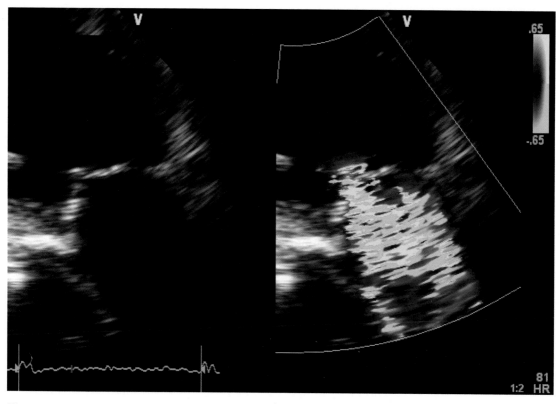

**Figure 3.1 Restricted posterior mitral leaflet.** Abnormal stresses on the inferior mitral leaflet as a result of an inferior or posterior myocardial infarct cause systolic restriction of the posterior leaflet (left), 'asymmetric tenting', with a posteriorly directed jet of regurgitation (right).

 And here's an electronic link to a loop on the website or use
http://goo.gl/B5IO2h

 And here's an electronic link to a loop on the website or use
http://goo.gl/txLqiv

**Table 3.3** Complications after myocardial infarction

| |
|---|
| Thrombus (Table 16.6, page 185) |
| True aneurysm (Figure 3.2a) |
| False aneurysm (Figure 3.2b) |
| Mitral regurgitation (Table 3.2) |

*(continued)*

**Table 3.3** Complications after myocardial infarction (*continued*)

| |
|---|
| Papillary muscle rupture |
| Ventricular septal rupture |
| Pericarditis* |
| Arrhythmia* |

*Not dependent on echocardiography for diagnosis

- If there is a murmur, check for mitral regurgitation and ventricular septal rupture. These may occasionally coexist. If there is mitral regurgitation, consider the causes in Table 3.2.
- Off-axis views may be necessary. An apical ventricular septal rupture in the presence of a small infarct may initially be obvious from abnormal systolic flow at the RV apex.
- Complete or partial rupture of the papillary muscle or septal rupture should be reported immediately to the responsible clinician.
- A true aneurysm complicates about 5% of all anterior infarcts and is a sign of a poor prognosis. It must be distinguished from a false aneurysm caused by free wall rupture contained by the pericardium (Table 3.4) (Figure 3.2).

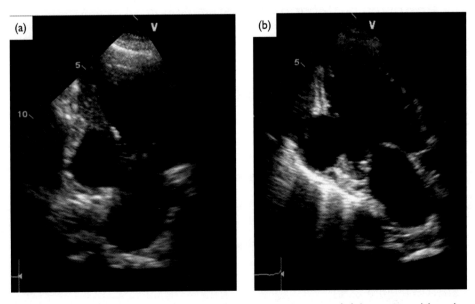

**Figure 3.2 True and false aneurysm.** A true aneurysm (a) is caused by the infarct bulging outwards so that there is a wide neck and the myocardium is often seen in the border-zone of the aneurysm. A false aneurysm (b) is a rupture of the infarcted myocardial wall with blood contained by the pericardium so that the false aneurysm contains no myocardial tissue.

And here's an electronic link to a loop on the website or use
http://goo.gl/wvoGQ4

Table 3.4 Differentiation of true and false aneurysms

|  | True aneurysm (Figure 3.2a) | False aneurysm (Figure 3.2b) |
|---|---|---|
| Position | More commonly apical | More commonly inferoposterior |
| Neck | Commonly wide | May be narrow |
| Boundaries | Myocardium | Pericardium |
| Colour flow | Usually absent | Into in systole, out in diastole |

- Occasionally a true aneurysm leaks and is associated with a false aneurysm.
- Sometimes an aneurysm is found in the absence of an acute history. The differential diagnosis is given in Table 3.5.

Table 3.5 Differential diagnosis of apical aneurysm as a presenting feature

| |
|---|
| Coronary disease |
| Syphilis |
| Chagas disease |
| Iatrogenic (e.g. surgical vent) |
| Congenital |
| Tuberculosis |
| Hypertropic cardiomyopathy (see pages 32–36) |

## 6 Consider stress echocardiography

Indications for stress echocardiography include:

- typical cardiac chest pain and normal or equivocal ECG changes and troponin levels
- minor or definite troponin rise but clinically stable and high risk from contrast angiography (e.g. renal failure)
- residual coronary stenosis in a non-culprit vessel and decision for intervention to be based on ischaemic burden.

# MISTAKES TO AVOID

- Failing to assess functional mitral regurgitation adequately
- Missing inferior wall motion abnormalities with incomplete views
- Missing a ventricular septal rupture by not using off-axis views if needed
- Not responding to a hyperdynamic LV which after a myocardial infarct may suggest a large ventricular septal rupture or severe mitral regurgitation

## CHECKLIST FOR REPORTING ACUTE CORONARY SYNDROME

1. LV size and function:
   a. Dimensions
   b. Regional wall motion
   c. Global systolic function
2. Right ventricle
3. Mitral valve appearance and regurgitation (if moderate or more, increases risk of events)
4. Complications:
   a. Thrombus
   b. True aneurysm
   c. False aneurysm
   d. Ventricular septal rupture
   e. Mitral regurgitation

## References

1. Prasad A, Lerman A, Rihal CS. Apical ballooning syndrome (Tako-Tsubo or stress cardiomyopathy): a mimic of acute myocardial infarction. *Am Heart J* 2008;155:408–17.
2. Ghadri JR, Ruschitzka F, Luscher TF, Templin C. Takotsubo cardiomyopathy: still much to learn. *Heart* 2014;100:1804–12.
3. Grigioni F, Enriquez-Sarano M, Zehr KJ, Bailey KR, Tajik AJ. Ischemic mitral regurgitation: long-term outcome and prognostic implications with quantitative Doppler assessment. *Circulation* 2001;103:1759–64.

# Cardiomyopathies

## 4

- Cardiomyopathies are muscle diseases not caused by coronary, valve or congenital disease or by systemic hypertension.
- They may be caused by primary familial muscle disease, by infiltrative processes (e.g. amyloid), storage diseases or by external agents (e.g. alcohol, radiation, anthracyclines).
- Their diagnosis is based on a balance of clinical factors (presentation, family history, past history, examination), the ECG findings and imaging.
- Echocardiography is the first-line imaging technique and provides an initial categorisation into:
  - dilated LV including idiopathic dilated cardiomyopathy
  - hypertrophied LV including hypertrophic cardiomyopathy.
- Other cardiomyopathies also have characteristic echocardiographic features:
  - restrictive cardiomyopathy – non-dilated with biatrial enlargement
  - noncompaction – hypertrabeculation
  - arrhythmogenic ventricular cardiomyopathy – RV dilatation.

## The dilated left ventricle

Secondary myocardial impairment and cardiomyopathies may look similar on echocardiography, but there may still be clues to the aetiology (Table 4.1).

Table 4.1 Causes of a dilated, hypokinetic left ventricle

| Cause | Notes |
|---|---|
| **Common** | |
| Coronary disease | Typically regional wall abnormalities or scarring although the hypokinesis may be global |
| Hypertension | Often thick-wall LV and other associations, e.g. dilated aorta and thickened aortic valve |
| Alcohol | May recover after alcohol cessation in 50% |
| HIV | Occurs in 10% of all asymptomatic cases |

(*continued*)

Table 4.1 Causes of a dilated, hypokinetic left ventricle (*continued*)

| Cause | Notes |
|---|---|
| End-stage aortic valve disease or mitral regurgitation | Differentiating secondary from primary mitral regurgitation may be difficult (see Chapter 8 and Table 4.5) |
| Tachyarrhythmia | Uncontrolled persistent atrial tachyarrhythmia or occasionally very frequent VPC |
| Nutritional | Deficiencies of thiamine, carnitine or selenium |
| Drugs | Verapamil, chemotherapeutic agents |
| Renal failure | Multifactorial including underlying disease, anaemia and uraemia |
| **Uncommon** | |
| Myocarditis | Viral, systemic lupus erythematosus (SLE) and other vasculitides including Kawasaki. Wall thickness may be increased in acute myocarditis especially in giant cell myocarditis |
| Peripartum cardiomyopathy | Occurs in the last month of pregnancy and up to the first 5 months after delivery |
| Neuromuscular disorders | Duchennes, Beckers and Emery–Dreifus (see Table 18.8, pages 201–2) |
| Familial dilated cardiomyopathies | Family history of heart failure, cardiomyopathy or sudden death |
| Sarcoid | Thinning and dilatation crossing arterial territories |
| Haemochromatosis | Diastolic dysfunction occurs early and LV dilatation late |
| Cocaine | Acute or chronic use |
| Endocrine | Hypothyroidism, diabetes, phaeochromocytoma |

# 1 Categorise by cavity dimensions and systolic function

- Some normal ranges in use are too narrow and may result in overdiagnosis of left ventricular dilatation, especially in large subjects. Diastolic diameters as large as 59 mm may be normal in large individuals (see Table 2.1).
- Is the left ventricle hypokinetic (Table 4.1), normal or hyperkinetic (Table 4.2)? Borderline hypokinesis is normal in athletic hearts (Table 4.3).

Table 4.2 Causes of a dilated, hyperkinetic left ventricle

| Valve lesions |
| --- |
| Severe aortic regurgitation |
| Severe mitral regurgitation |
| Moderate or worse mixed aortic and mitral regurgitation |
| **Shunts** |
| Persistent ductus |
| Ventricular septal defect |
| Ruptured sinus of valsalva aneurysm |

Table 4.3 Features of an athletic heart[1]

| |
| --- |
| Left ventricular dilatation: diastolic diameter up to 70 mm in men and 66 mm in women |
| Normal systolic function, occasionally borderline global hypokinesis |
| Mild left ventricular hypertrophy, septum usually ≤13 mm |
| Normal LV diastolic function |
| Mild RV dilatation and hypertrophy |

## 2 General appearance

- Is there a regional abnormality suggesting an ischaemic aetiology (see Figure 2.3)?
- Is there concentric LV hypertrophy suggesting hypertension?
- Are both ventricles dilated suggesting a cardiomyopathy?
- Is there a valve abnormality which might have caused the myocardial impairment?
- Are there unusual features?
  - Regional wall motion abnormality crossing arterial territories (e.g. sarcoid) (Table 4.4)
  - Bright endocardial echoes (e.g. haemochromatosis)
  - Apical echogenicity (consider thrombus, hypertrophic cardiomyopathy or noncompaction)
  - Abnormal myocardial density (non-specific but consider amyloid)

**Table 4.4** Echocardiographic findings in sarcoid[2]

| |
|---|
| Regional wall thinning especially at base of heart |
| Aneurysmal dilatation |
| Occasionally global LV dysfunction |
| Localised mass (may involve papillary muscle causing mitral regurgitation) |
| Pericardial effusion |

# 3 Quantify systolic function and assess diastolic function

See pages 12–18.

# 4 Are there complications?

- LV thrombus
- Secondary mitral regurgitation (Table 4.5)
- Pulmonary hypertension

**Table 4.5** Differentiating primary and secondary mitral regurgitation with a dilated LV

| **Favours secondary regurgitation** |
|---|
| Mitral valve normal in appearance |
| Mitral valve tented |
| Review of echocardiograms shows LV function declining while mitral regurgitation absent or still mild |
| **Favours primary regurgitation** |
| Mitral valve abnormal in appearance e.g., rheumatic or prolapsing |
| Review of echocardiograms shows severe mitral regurgitation with previously hyperdynamic LV |

# 5 Other imaging modalities

- **Cardiac magnetic resonance (CMR)[3, 4]:**
  - Differentiation of ischaemia from other causes of LV dilatation by the pattern of late gadolinium enhancement (transmural, patchy subendocardial, global subendocardial, epicardial, midwall)
  - Assessment of viability in ischaemic cardiomyopathy.

- Better than echocardiography for LV morphology, volumes and ejection fraction if image quality suboptimal
- May help in the diagnosis of myocarditis using T2-weighted oedema imaging as a tool for evaluating myocardial inflammation and early and late gadolinium enhancement to assess diseased myocardium
- May help in the diagnosis of myocarditis, especially of giant cell myocarditis
- T2* imaging detects and quantifies iron deposits in the myocardium in haemochromatosis
- Detection of aneurysms in Chagas disease
- **Computerised tomography (CT) coronary angiography:** to look for coronary disease as a cause of LV dilatation, especially in patients at low clinical risk of coronary disease
- **Invasive contrast coronary angiography:** to look for coronary disease as a cause of LV dilatation, especially in patients at high or intermediate risk of coronary disease
- **Positron emission tomography (PET):** mismatch between fluorodeoxyglucose (FDG) and ammonia may identify myocardial viability

 ## MISTAKES TO AVOID

- Cutting LV obliquely especially using M-mode causing overdiagnosis of LV dilatation
- Overdiagnosis of dilatation by not correcting for BSA in large individuals
- Misdiagnosis of athletes heart as cardiomyopathy
- Mistaking LV dilatation as a result of primary mitral valve disease as a cardiomyopathy

## CHECKLIST FOR REPORTING LV DILATATION

1. LV dimensions, wall thickness and morphology (including trabeculation)
2. LV regional and global systolic and diastolic function
3. RV size and function
4. Pulmonary pressure
5. Valve function – as a cause of LV dilatation but also secondary mitral regurgitation as a complication
6. LV thrombus?

# The hypertrophied left ventricle

- The cause of LV hypertrophy may be obvious if there is aortic stenosis or systemic hypertension.
- Often it may be difficult to differentiate the effects of hypertension from an athletic heart or hypertrophic cardiomyopathy or less common causes (Table 4.6).

Table 4.6 Causes of increased LV wall thickness[5, 6]

| Common |
|---|
| Hypertension |
| Aortic stenosis |
| Obesity |
| Athleticism (usually mild hypertrophy) |
| **Cardiomyopathies** |
| Hypertrophic cardiomyopathies |
| Infiltrative diseases (e.g amyloid) |
| Glycogen storage diseases (e.g. Pompe's, Forbe's, Danon) |
| Lysosomal storage diseases (e.g. Anderson-Fabry, Hurler's) |
| Syndromic HCM (Friedrich's ataxia, Noonan, LEOPARD) |

## 1 Describe the pattern of hypertrophy

- Is it symmetrical or asymmetrical and does it affect RV as well as LV (Table 4.7)?
- Asymmetric hypertrophy suggests HCM. Describe its distribution, for example:
  - apical (Figure 4.1)
  - septum alone
  - septum and free wall, sparing the posterior wall
  - subaortic alone. This may be normal in an elderly person but may be the first site of hypertrophy associated with hypertension. If severe and in a young person, it may also be consistent with HCM.

Table 4.7 Patterns of hypertrophy

| Pattern | Suggestive diagnoses |
|---|---|
| Symmetrical | Storage and infiltrative disorders |
| Asymmetrical | HCM |
| Affects both ventricles | Storage and infiltrative disorders |

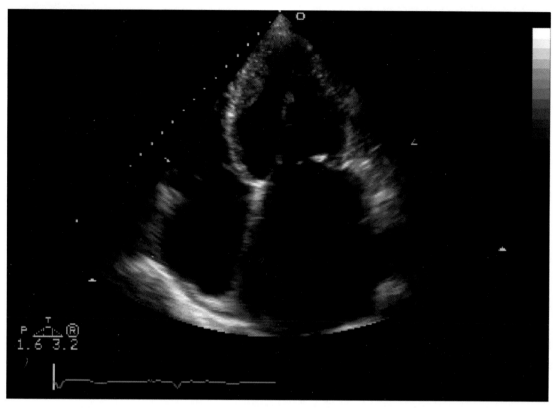

**Figure 4.1 Apical hypertrophic cardiomyopathy.**

## 2 If the hypertrophy is asymmetric, measure wall thickness at all levels

- Measure representative thicknesses at base and mid segment usually in the parasternal short-axis (PSAX) view depending on the pattern of hypertrophy: anterior, posterior, lateral and septum.
- A wall thickness ≥30 mm in any segment is a strong marker for sudden death in HCM.

## 3 Quantify systolic function and assess diastolic function

- Impaired systolic function with significant hypertrophy suggests amyloid rather than hypertrophic cardiomyopathy.
- A reduced EF <50% in HCM indicates a high risk of sudden death.
- Restrictive rather than slow or pseudonormal filling suggests amyloid cardiomyopathy.

# 4 Is there an apical aneurysm?

- This is uncommon in HCM but indicates a high risk of sudden death.[7]
- It may require contrast echocardiography or sometimes CMR if image quality is suboptimal.

# 5 Measure LA size

- LA dilatation is multifactorial in origin (presence of MR, LV diastolic dysfunction, atrial myopathy).
- Severe LA dilatation (see page 141) is associated with severe disease and poor outcome with a threshold >34 ml/m$^2$ in one study.[8]

# 6 Assess the valves

Look for the following:
- Systolic anterior motion of the anterior leaflet of the mitral valve or of the chordae alone
- Mitral regurgitation directed posteriorly away from the point of anterior motion
- Abnormal mitral valve appearance:
  - abnormally long anterior leaflet may occur in HCM
  - mitral valve thickening from septal contact
  - mitral prolapse
  - evidence of previous endocarditis (HCM is a risk factor)
- Early closure of the aortic valve (associated with dynamic LV outflow acceleration)
- Severe aortic stenosis or subaortic membrane as an alternative cause of LV hypertrophy

# 7 Is there intracavitary or outflow tract flow acceleration?

- This is assessed using continuous wave Doppler from the apex. On the first visit it should be assessed at rest and after valsalva performed supine then sitting and, if no gradient is provoked, on standing.[9]
- Differentiate a fixed obstruction (peaking in early or mid-systole) and a late systolic peak from systolic anterior motion of the mitral valve in HCM.
- A peak velocity ≥2.7 m/s (30 mmHg) indicates a relatively high risk of death related to HCM[10] but not of sudden death. A peak velocity ≥3.5 m/s (gradient 50 mmHg) is the threshold for intervention.
- In patients with symptoms and resting or provoked LV outflow tract velocity <3.5 m/s (<50 mmHg), exercise testing is indicated[9, 11] to look for acceleration ≥3.5 m/s as an indication for considering myomectomy.

## 8 Hypertrophic cardiomyopathy vs hypertension

- The diagnosis of a cardiomyopathy is made using all available clinical data.
- The echocardiography report alone should never make a new diagnosis, but can suggest HCM (Table 4.8).

## 9 Hypertrophic cardiomyopathy vs athletic heart

- Endurance or resistance training usually causes an increase in cavity size but only mild septal thickening (≤13 mm) (Table 4.9).
- Endurance athletes have larger cavity volumes than resistance athletes but wall thickness is similar.[12]

Table 4.8 Features in favour of hypertrophic cardiomyopathy rather than hypertensive disease

| |
|---|
| Localised hypertrophy most frequently affecting the septum |
| Hypertrophy affecting both ventricles |
| Septal hypertrophy ≥15mm (Caucasian) and ≥20 mm (Afro-Caribbean) |
| Abnormally long anterior mitral leaflet |
| Severe systolic anterior motion of the anterior mitral leaflet |
| Severe intracavitary flow acceleration |
| Severe diastolic dysfunction |
| No regression after blood pressure control |
| Large QRS voltages and T wave changes on the ECG |

Table 4.9 Features in favour of cardiomyopathy rather than athletic heart[13]

| |
|---|
| LV cavity dimension <45 mm |
| Significant LA enlargement |
| Diastolic dysfunction |
| Female gender or family history of hypertrophic cardiomyopathy |
| Abnormal ECG |
| No change with detraining |

## 10 Hypertrophic cardiomyopathy vs storage or infiltrative disorders

Any pattern can occur in HCM but the features in Table 4.10 favour storage or infiltrative disorders.

Table 4.10 Features favouring storage (e.g. Anderson-Fabry) or infiltration (e.g. amyloid) rather than hypertrophic cardiomyopathy[5]

| |
|---|
| Symmetric rather than asymmetric LV hypertrophy |
| LV hypokinesis |
| Associated RV hypertrophy |
| Small complexes on ECG (amyloid) |
| Valve thickening in 15% with Fabry[14] |

## 11 Other imaging modalities

- **CMR**[3] may be used to:
  - improve the description of the hypertrophy, particularly looking for RV involvement and apical LV involvement
  - identify apical aneurysms
  - detect and quantify myocardial fibrosis
  - exclude differential diagnoses (amyloid, Anderson-Fabry).

 **MISTAKES TO AVOID**

- Over-reporting a normal subaortic septal bulge in the elderly
- Making a new diagnosis of HCM from the echo alone. This is a clinical diagnosis
- Mistaking mitral regurgitation for the LV outflow jet on continuous wave Doppler
- Missing a subaortic membrane as a cause of non-valvar LV outflow acceleration and LV hypertrophy

## CHECKLIST FOR REPORTING LV HYPERTROPHY

1. Location of hypertrophy (check RV as well)
2. Wall thickness at representative levels
3. LV systolic and diastolic function
4. Systolic anterior motion and LV outflow acceleration?
5. Are there echocardiographic risk factors for death (Septal width $\geq$30 mm, reduced EF, outflow acceleration $\geq$2.7 m/s)?

# Restrictive cardiomyopathy

- In a patient suspected of heart failure with no obvious LV hypertrophy or dilatation, restrictive cardiomyopathy is defined by:
  - restrictive LV filling
  - normal or slightly reduced LV cavity size
  - normal or mildly reduced LV systolic function.
- The causes include infiltrative (e.g. amyloid) and storage disorders, endocardial pathology (endomyocardial fibrosis, carcinoid) and familial or acquired myocardial pathology (anthracycline) (Table 4.11).
- An important differential diagnosis is pericardial constriction since pericardial thickening may be associated with involvement of the epicardial myocardium, e.g. after irradiation. These are differentiated on pages 175–176.

Table 4.11 Restrictive cardiomyopathies

| Cardiomyopathy | Comment |
|---|---|
| Amyloid | Table 4.10 |
| Scleroderma | Uncommon, usually subclinical. Associated thickening of skin |
| Post-irradiation | Valve thickening. Combined constriction |
| Carcinoid | Characteristic tricuspid or pulmonary valve thickening |
| Haemachromatosis | Endocardial echogenicity |
| Glycogen storage | e.g. Pompe's |
| Lysosomal storage diseases | e.g. Anderson-Fabry's |
| Drugs | e.g. Anthracyclines |
| Endomyocardial fibrosis | Table 4.12 |
| Endomyocardial diseases with eosinophilia | Table 4.12 |
| Idiopathic | Diagnosis by exclusion |

Table 4.12 Features of endomyocardial fibrosis diseases

| |
|---|
| Echogenicity at RV or LV apex (Figure 4.2) |
| Subvalvar LV or RV thickening |
| Tricuspid or mitral regurgitation |
| LV or RV thrombus |

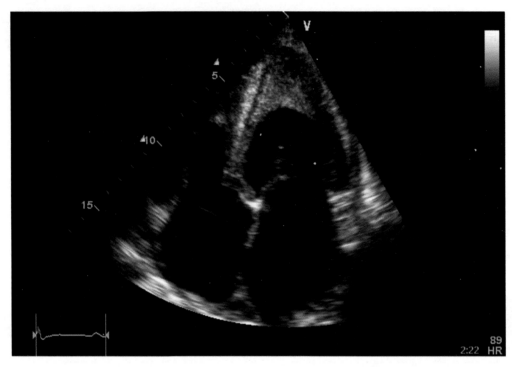

**Figure 4.2 Endomyocardial fibrosis.** There is thrombosis at the apex of both left and right ventricle.

 And here's an electronic link to a loop on the website or use
http://goo.gl/hA9Ueh

## Other techniques

- **CMR:**
  - T2* imaging for assessing myocardial iron content in patients receiving multiple blood transfusions and haemachromatosis
  - abnormal myocardial and blood-pool gadolinium kinetics are seen with amyloidosis.
- **99mTc-DPD scintigraphy** may be used for the detection of amyloidosis.

 ## MISTAKES TO AVOID

- Mistaking the presence of restrictive physiology for restrictive cardiomyopathy. Restrictive physiology occurs in any situation with a high-filling pressure and rapid cessation of flow (e.g. post myocardial infarction, pericardial constriction)

**CHECKLIST FOR REPORTING RESTRICTIVE CARDIOMYOPATHY**

1. LV size and systolic function
2. LV diastolic function
3. Valve appearance and function
4. If pericardial constriction is a possible diagnosis (pages 172–176), measure:
   - respiratory variability of transmitral and subaortic flow
   - IVC size and response to respiration

# Noncompaction

- The foetal heart is heavily trabeculated but becomes compacted during development. Noncompaction arises from either interruption of this process or the new growth of trabeculation later in life.
- New trabeculation can occur in other cardiomyopathies (dilated or hypertrophic), or with physiological stimuli (e.g. exercise training) or may occur as a separate pathological entity.
- The presentation is classically with heart failure, ventricular arrhythmia or systemic emboli, but the diagnosis may be made on family screening.
- The echocardiogram shows numerous (>3) prominent trabeculations (Figure 4.3) (Table 4.13):
   - Approximately how many trabeculations are there (<3, 3–5, or many)?
   - Describe the site of the trabeculations (apex, inferior, lateral wall).
   - Show on colour mapping that flow penetrates to the bases of the recesses (consider transpulmonary contrast).
   - A ratio of trabeculation:underlying wall >2 fulfills the commonly used Jenni criteria.[15]
   - Look for thrombus in the recesses.
- Assess the LV. Systolic function is often reduced.
- Look for other congenital cardiac abnormalities.
- The differential for hypertrabeculation[16] is:

   - trabeculation associated with athletic training especially in Afro-Caribbean athletes
   - normal trabeculation
   - trabeculation in hypertrophic cardiomyopathy
   - trabeculation in dilated or peripartum cardiomyopathy
   - false tendons.

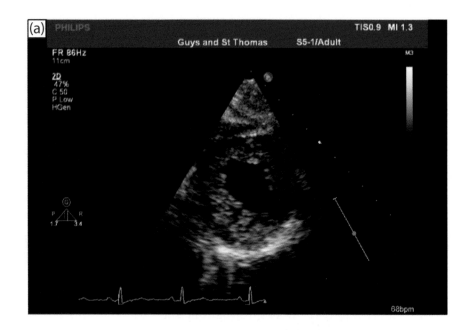

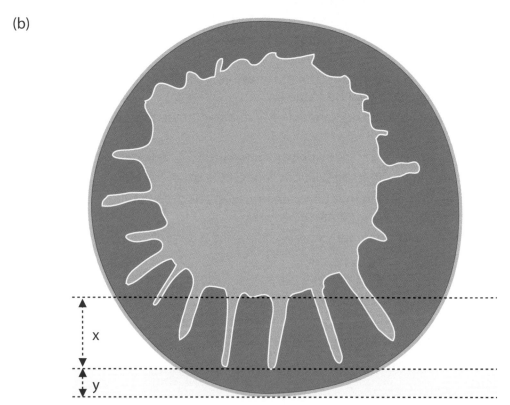

Figure 4.3 Noncompaction. A parasternal short-axis view showing posterior trabeculation (a) is illustrated diagrammatically in (b). Measure the average length of trabeculation and the underlying normal wall in a short-axis end-systolic frame. A ratio of trabeculation:underlying wall (x:y) >2 fulfills the commonly used Jenni diagnostic criteria.[14]

**Table 4.13** Features of isolated ventricular noncompaction[15, 17]

| Features |
|---|
| >3 large trabeculae (usually at apex, mid-inferior or free wall) with deep intratrabecular recesses (confirmed on colour mapping) |
| Ratio of noncompacted (trabeculae) to compacted (underlying muscle) >2 on an end-systolic parasternal short-axis view (Figure 4.3) |
| Absence of congenital causes of pressure-load (e.g. LV outflow obstruction) |
| **Associated features** |
| Hypokinesis of affected segments |
| Dilatation and hypokinesis of unaffected segments usually at the base of the LV |
| Abnormal ECG (LBBB, Poor R wave progression, pathological Q waves) |

# Arrhythmogenic right ventricular cardiomyopathy/dysplasia

- The diagnosis of arrhythmogenic right ventricular cardiomyopathy/dysplasia (ARVC/D) is based on a combination of histology, imaging (echo and magnetic resonance), electrocardiographic depolarisation and repolarisation abnormalities, arrhythmias and family history.
- On echocardiography there must be regional akinesis, dyskinesis (not hypokinesis) or aneurysms (Figure 4.4) and RV dilatation (Table 4.14) (Figure 4.5).
- RV function is quantified within the guidelines by percentage area change.
- LV involvement is common (and may sometimes dominate over RV involvement).
- The differential diagnosis of a dilated hypokinetic RV is:
  - RV infarct
  - dilated cardiomyopathy confined to the RV
  - pulmonary hypertension
  - ARVC/D.

**Table 4.14** Echocardiographic features of arrhythmogenic RV cardiomyopathy/dysplasia in addition to RV akinesis, dyskinesis or aneurysms[18]

| Major criteria | |
|---|---|
| PLAX RVOT | $\geq$32 mm ($\geq$19 mm/m$^2$) |
| PSAX RVOT | $\geq$36 mm ($\geq$21 mm/m$^2$) |
| RV fractional area change* | $\leq$33% |

(*continued*)

**Table 4.14** Echocardiographic features of arrhythmogenic RV cardiomyopathy/ dysplasia (*continued*)

| Minor criteria | |
|---|---|
| PLAX RVOT | ≥29 mm (≥16≤18 mm/m²) |
| PSAX RVOT | ≥32 mm (≥18≤20 mm/m²) |
| RV fractional area change | ≤40% |

PLAX RVOT: parasternal long-axis RV outflow tract; PSAX RVOT: parasternal short-axis RV outflow tract
*Measured by tracing the RV endocardium in systole and diastole in the 4-chamber view. Subtract the systolic area from the diastolic area and divide by the diastolic area. Multiplying by 100 expresses the difference as a percentage

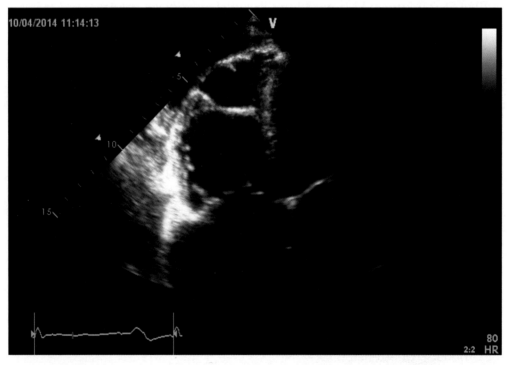

**Figure 4.4 ARVC/D.** Zoomed apical 4-chamber view of a dilated right ventricle to show aneurysms.

## Other imaging modalities

- **CMR:**
  - Noncompaction: CMR may be useful especially if echocardiographic image quality is suboptimal. The diagnosis is suggested with a noncompaction: compacted ratio >2.3 at end diastole.
  - ARVC/D: CMR is useful for assessing RV size and morphology and for detecting subclinical left ventricular involvement.

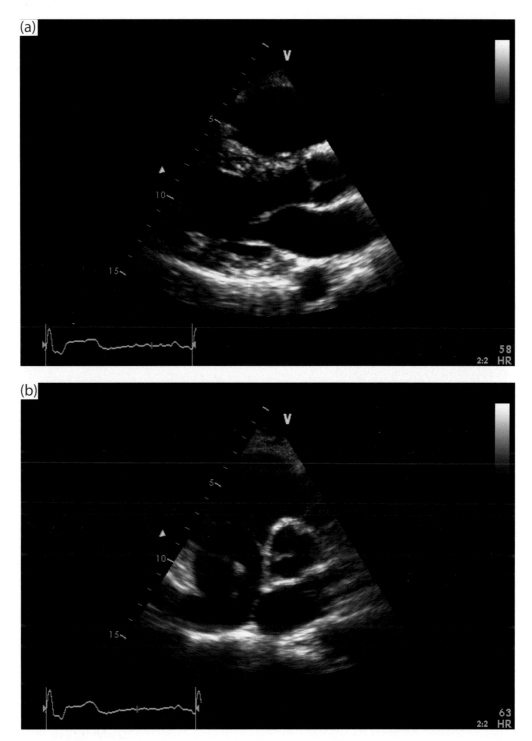

**Figure 4.5 ARVC/D.** (a) Parasternal long-axis view showing an enlarged RV outflow tract diameter at 44 mm, and (b) parasternal short-axis view showing an RV outflow tract diameter is 37 mm.

## CHECKLIST FOR REPORTING NONCOMPACTION AND ARVC/D

**Noncompaction**

1. Number of trabeculations
2. Site of trabeculation
3. Length of trabeculation compared to compacted myocardium
4. LV systolic and diastolic function
5. Exclude other congenital anomalies
6. Complications, e.g. thrombus, mitral regurgitation

**ARVC/D**

1. RV regional akinesis or dyskinesis or aneurysms?
2. RV dimensions
3. RV fractional area change
4. Exclude pulmonary hypertension and other causes of RV dilatation (Table 5.2, page 48)
5. LV size and systolic function

## References

1. Fagard R. Athlete's heart. *Heart* 2003;89(12):1455–61.
2. Doughan AR, Williams BR. Cardiac sarcoidosis. *Heart* 2006;92(2):282–8.
3. To ACY, Dhillon A, Desai MY. Cardiac magnetic resonance in hypertrophic cardiomyopathy. *JACC Cardiovasc Imaging* 2011;4:1123–37.
4. Marques JS, Pinto FJ. Clinical use of multimodality imaging in the assessment of dilated cardiomyopathy. *Heart* 2015;101:562–72.
5. Elliott P, Andersson B, Arbustini E et al. Classification of the cardiomyopathies: a position statement from the European Society of Cardiology Working Group on Cardiomyopathies, Myocardial and Pericardial Diseases. *Eur Heart J* 2008;29:270–6.
6. Schunkert H. Echocardiographic and hemodynamic data in obese patients. *Heart Metab* 2002;17:15–20.
7. Maron MS, Finley JJ, Bos JM et al. Prevalence, clinical significance, and natural history of left ventricular apical aneurysms in hypertrophic cardiomyopathy. *Circulation* 2008;118:1541–9.
8. Yang H, Woo A, Monakier D et al. Enlarged left atrial volume in hypertrophic cardiomyopathy: a marker for disease severity. *J Am Soc Echocardiogr* 2005;18:1074–82.
9. Elliott PM, Anastasakis A, Borger MA et al. 2014 ESC guidelines on diagnosis and management of hypertrophic cardiomyopathy. *Eur Heart J* 2014;35:2733–79.

10. Maron MS, Olivotto I, Betocchi S et al. Effect of left ventricular outflow tract obstruction on clinical outcome in hypertrophic cardiomyopathy. *N Engl J Med* 2003;348:295–303.
11. Nagueh SF, Bierig SM, Budoff MJ et al. American Society of Echocardiography recommendations for multimodality cardiovascular imaging of patients with hypertrophic cardiomyopathy. *J Am Soc Echocardiogr* 2011;24:473–98.
12. Utomi V, Oxborough D, Whyte GP et al. Systematic review and meta-analysis of training mode, imaging modality and body size influences on the morphology and function of the male athlete's heart. *Heart* 2013;99:1727–33.
13. Maron BJ. Distinguishing hypertrophic cardiomyopathy from athlete's heart: a clinical problem of increasing magnitude and significance. *Heart* 2005;91(11):1380-2.
14. Linhart A, Kampmann C, Zamorano JL et al. Cardiac manifestations of Andersen-Fabry disease: results from the International Fabry outcome survey. *Eur Heart J* 2007;28:1228–35.
15. Jenni R, Oechslin E, Schneider J, Attenhofer JC, Kaufmann PA. Echocardiographic and pathoanatomical characteristics of isolated left ventricular non-compaction: a step towards classification as a distinct cardiomyopathy. *Heart* 2001;86(6):666-71.
16. Stollberger C, Finsterer J. Pitfalls in the diagnosis of left ventricular hypertrabeculation/non-compaction. *Postgrad Med J* 2006;82:679–83.
17. Almeida AG, Pinto FJ. Non-compaction cardiomyopathy. *Heart* 2013;99:1535–42.
18. Marcus FI, McKenna WJ, Sherill D et al. Diagnosis of arrhythmogenic right ventricular cardiomyopathy/dysplasia. Proposed modifications of the Task Force criteria. *Circulation* 2010;121:1533–41.

# The right ventricle

## 5

Measurement of RV size is part of the minimum standard study. A more detailed assessment is required if there is:

- RV dilatation on the initial study
- congenital heart disease
- severe left-sided valve disease
- right-sided valve disease
- suspected RV cardiomyopathy
- pulmonary hypertension
- suspected pulmonary embolism
- chronic lung disease
- cardiac transplantation.

## 1 Is the RV dilated?

- Use views optimised for the right ventricle.
- As a guide, significant dilatation is present if the RV is the same size or larger than the normal LV in the apical 4-chamber view.
- If the RV is dilated, three diameters should be measured as shown in Figure 5.1. Normal values for these are given in Table 5.1.

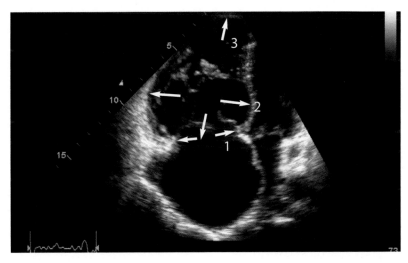

**Figure 5.1 Levels for measuring RV size.** 1 is at the annulus, 2 is the maximum transverse diameter, and 3 is base-to-apex. This is a 4-chamber view centred on the right ventricle in a patient with arrhythmogenic RV dysplasia.

Table 5.1 Upper limit of normal RV dimensions, measured in diastole (mm)[1]

| Right ventricle dimension | Measurement in diastole (mm) |
|---|---|
| Basal (RVD1) | 42 |
| Mid (RVD2) | 35 |
| Length base to apex (RVD3) | 86 |

## 2 If large, is the RV active or hypokinetic?

- An active RV suggests a left-to-right shunt or tricuspid or pulmonary regurgitation (Table 5.2).
- A hypokinetic right ventricle suggests pulmonary hypertension, myocardial infarction or a myopathy (Table 5.2).
- Look for a regional abnormality of contraction and also check the inferior wall of the LV since about a third of inferior LV infarcts are associated with RV infarction.

Table 5.2 Causes of right ventricular dilatation

| Active RV |
|---|
| Left to right shunt above the right ventricle (i.e. ASD) |
| Tricuspid or pulmonary regurgitation |
| **Hypokinetic RV** |
| Pulmonary hypertension especially acute pulmonary embolism |
| Right ventricular infarction |
| Right ventricular myopathy |
| End-stage pulmonary valve disease or tricuspid regurgitation |

## 3 Quantification of systolic function using long-axis measurements

- Tricuspid annular plane systolic excursion (TAPSE). Place the M-mode cursor on the junction between the RV free wall and tricuspid annulus in a zoomed 4-chamber view. Measure the excursion as the vertical distance between the peak and nadir (Figure 5.2). The threshold for impaired function is 16 mm.[1]
- Tissue Doppler imaging (TDI). Place a pulsed Doppler tissue sample in the RV free wall just above the tricuspid annulus ensuring good alignment (Table 5.3). Record the peak systolic velocity. The threshold for abnormality is a systolic velocity (S or S1) <10 cm/s.[1]

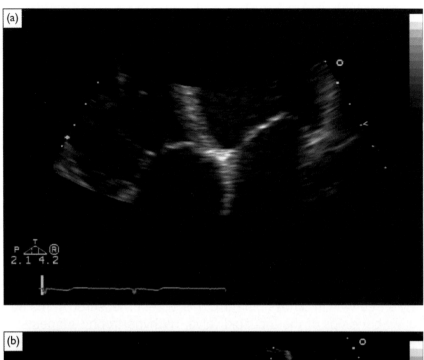

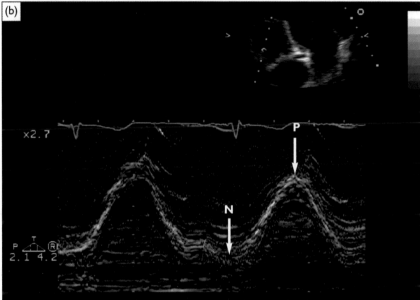

**Figure 5.2 Long-axis excursion.** Position for placing the M-mode cursor and the M-mode recording obtained. Excursion is measured between the nadir (N) and peak (P).

Table 5.3 Thresholds for abnormal RV function[1]

| Measurement | Threshold |
| --- | --- |
| TAPSE (mm) | <16 |
| Tissue Doppler systolic velocity (cm/s) | <10 |
| MPI (if measured)* | <0.55 |
| RV d$P$/d$t$ (mmHg/s)† | <400 |

*Myocardial performance index (also called the Tei index)
†Measure the time interval in seconds between 1 m/s and 2 m/s of the downstroke of the TR waveform and divide into 12. Note that this involves a different calculation to that used for LV d$P$/d$t$ when using the MR jet. The measurement is not recommended for routine use but may help if there is uncertainty about RV function

## 4 Is there right ventricular hypertrophy?

- Defined by a free wall thickness >5 mm. This is best measured in the subcostal view level with the tips of the tricuspid valve. RV hypertrophy suggests:
  - Eisenmenger syndrome (pulmonary hypertension as a result of left-to-right shunting)
  - pulmonary stenosis
  - storage disease
  - amyloid
  - hypertrophic cardiomyopathy.

## 5 Is there left-sided disease?

- RV dilatation as a result of pulmonary hypertension may complicate severe mitral stenosis, but it can also occur in end-stage aortic stenosis or mitral regurgitation or severe LV dysfunction.

## 6 Is there evidence of a shunt above the right ventricle?

- If the RV is dilated and active, but no ASD is visible, injection of agitated saline may show an ASD as a void caused by a left-to-right jet or by the right-to-left passage of 'bubbles'.
- Otherwise consider transoesophageal echocardiography (TOE), which is usually necessary to detect a sinus venosus defect or partial anomalous pulmonary venous drainage.

## 7 Is there tricuspid and pulmonary regurgitation?

See pages 95 and 102.

## 8 Estimate pulmonary artery pressure

See pages 53–54.

## 9 Other techniques

CMR is the gold-standard technique for assessing RV volumes and should be considered for serial studies in patients with severe pulmonary regurgitation to guide intervention.

 **MISTAKES TO AVOID**

- When making RV measurements in the apical views, align the right heart so that it is in the centre of the image sector. Avoid foreshortening by scanning from a rib space too high as this can lead to overestimating the transverse diameters.
- Avoid including fat when measuring RV wall thickness.
- Do not use colour-coded TDI to measure the RV S wave because the values are lower than using pulsed tissue Doppler and there are no established normal ranges.

**CHECKLIST FOR REPORTING THE RIGHT VENTRICLE**

1. RV size and systolic function
2. Pulmonary pressures
3. Right-sided valve disease
4. Evidence of a shunt
5. Presence of left-sided disease

## References

1. Rudski L, Lai W, Afilalo J et al. Guidelines for the echocardiographic assessment of the right heart in adults: a report from the American Society of Echocardiography. *J Am Soc Echocardiogr* 2010;23:685-713.

# Pulmonary pressure and hypertension

## 6

## 1 Estimating right atrial pressure

- This is based on the diameter of the IVC (subcostal view) and response to sniffing (Table 6.1).
  - The diameter should be measured at end expiration close to the junction with the hepatic veins situated 0.5–3.0 cm from the ostium of the right atrium (RA).
  - During sniffing, avoid the IVC moving out of the imaging plane as this can exaggerate the reduction in diameter
  - In acutely ill patients in whom the subcostal view is suboptimal, a right anterior oblique midaxillary view can be used instead.[1]
- Estimating right atrial pressure is semi subjective. High and low pressures based on concordant IVC diameter and response to sniff are most secure (Table 6.1).

- If the IVC diameter and response to sniff is discordant (intermediate in Table 6.1):
  - assign as high if the IVC collapses <50%
  - assign as normal if there are no secondary indices (Table 6.2)
  - assign as intermediate if the IVC collapse is >50% but there are some secondary indices (Table 6.2).

Table 6.1 Estimating RA pressure[2]*

|  | Normal 0–5 mmHg (mean 3 mmHg) | Intermediate 5–10 mmHg (mean 8 mmHg) | | High 10–20 mmHg (mean 15 mmHg) |
|---|---|---|---|---|
| IVC diameter | ≤2.1 cm | ≤2.1 cm | >2.1 cm | >2.1 cm |
| Collapse with sniff | >50% | <50% | >50% | <50% |

*Either a range or a mean value may be used depending on local preference

Table 6.2 Secondary indices if the RA pressure estimate is intermediate

| |
|---|
| Restrictive right sided filling pattern (tricuspid E/A >2.1, deceleration time <120 ms) |
| Tricuspid E/E' >6 |
| Diastolic flow dominance in the hepatic vein |
| RA dilatation with no other cause e.g., TR, AF |
| Displacement of atrial septum to the left throughout the cycle |

## 2 Estimating PA systolic pressure

- Measure tricuspid regurgitant $V_{max}$. If the signal varies, take the highest value. Estimate the pressure difference ($4V^2$).
- Estimate the right atrial pressure (Tables 6.1 and 6.2).
- The sum of the transtricuspid and right atrial pressures gives the right ventricular systolic pressure. This is the same as pulmonary systolic pressure, assuming that there is no pulmonary stenosis or other RV outflow obstruction.

## 3 Estimating PA diastolic pressure

- Measure the end-diastolic velocity of the pulmonary regurgitant signal (Figure 6.1) and estimate the pressure difference ($4V^2$).
- Estimate the right atrial pressure (Tables 6.1 and 6.2).
- The sum of these is the pulmonary artery diastolic pressure.

## 4 Estimating PA mean pressure (if required)

- There are no firm methods so it is recommended that more than one is used:[3, 4]
  - ⅓PA systolic pressure + ⅔PA diastolic pressure
  - $4 \times PR\ V_{max}^2 + RA$ pressure

## 5 Detection of pulmonary hypertension if there is no measurable TR jet

- Pulmonary hypertension (PHT) still requires right heart catheterisation for a formal diagnosis and this also allows the assessment of pulmonary vascular resistance.
- If the TR signal is not analysable, the signal may be improved by bubble contrast.
- Alternatively, the PA systolic signal gives a guide to the presence of a raised systolic PA pressure (Figure 6.2).
  - Place the pulsed sample in the centre of the main pulmonary artery or the pulmonary valve annulus. Avoid placing the sample too near the artery wall which may give an artefactually sharp signal.
  - Measure the time from the start of flow to the peak velocity.
  - A time >105 ms excludes pulmonary hypertension[5] and <80 ms makes pulmonary hypertension highly likely. This method is not accurate enough to give an estimate of absolute pressure.
- The pulmonary regurgitant signal may indicate a raised diastolic or mean pressure (Figure 6.1, page 55).
- Other signs suggesting pulmonary hypertension are given in Table 6.3.

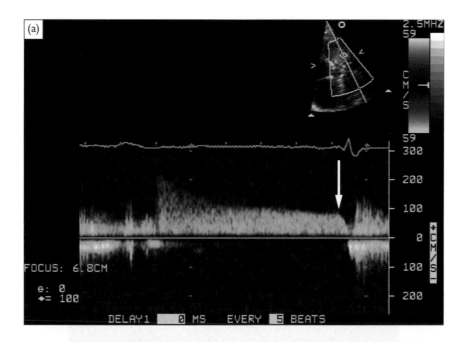

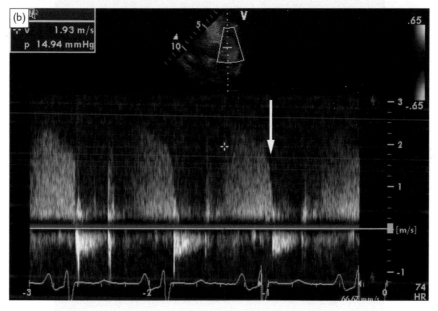

Figure 6.1 Pulmonary regurgitation. Pulmonary artery diastolic pressure is estimated using the end-diastolic velocity of the pulmonary regurgitant continuous wave signal (arrow) added to an estimate of right atrial pressure. (a) is a signal from a patient with normal pulmonary artery pressure and (b) a patient with pulmonary hypertension.

**Table 6.3** Signs suggesting pulmonary hypertension[2]

| TR $V_{max}$ >2.8–2.9* |
| --- |
| Estimated PA systolic pressure >35 mmHg |
| PA acceleration time <105 ms (more specific if <80 ms) |
| TAPSE <16 mm† |
| TDI pulsed <10 cm/s† |
| TDI colour <6 cm/s† |
| High early or end diastolic PR velocity |

*There is no simple single threshold; use all available echo modalities
†Assuming no RV infarction or myopathy

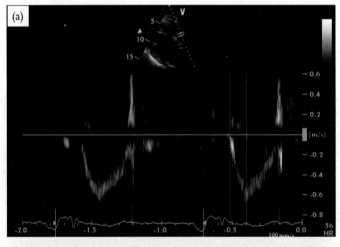

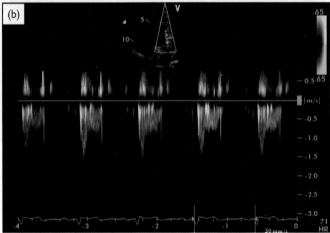

**Figure 6.2 Pulmonary artery velocity.** (a) A normal waveform with time to peak velocity 120 ms and (b) a recording in a patient with pulmonary hypertension. The time to peak velocity is short and the signal is notched as a result of increased wave reflectance.

# 6 Assess RV size and systolic function

See pages 47–50. Flattening of the interventricular septum in systole causing a D-shaped LV cavity is a clue that there could be pulmonary hypertension.

# 7 Assess the grade of tricuspid regurgitation

See page 96.

# 8 Look for causes of pulmonary hypertension

- The cardiac causes will be seen on echocardiography (Table 6.4).
- Other causes may be suggested on the echocardiogram by the presence of valve thickening or regurgitation (e.g. SLE, antiphospholipid syndrome, anorexic drugs) or aortic dilatation (e.g. rheumatoid arthritis).

Table 6.4 Cardiac causes of pulmonary hypertension detectable on echocardiography[6]

| **Pulmonary venous hypertension** |
| --- |
| Valve disease <br> • Mitral valve disease (stenosis > regurgitation) <br> • Severe aortic stenosis (pulmonary hypertension in at least 25%) |
| Severe left ventricular impairment <br> • Cardiomyopathy <br> • LV failure of any cause |
| Congenital heart disease without shunts <br> • Coarctation <br> • Subaortic or supravalvar stenosis |
| Pericardial constriction |
| Left atrial obstruction <br> • Myxoma <br> • Cor triatriatum |
| Pulmonary vein obstruction <br> • Congenital vein stenosis <br> • Mediastinal pathology (fibrosis, tumour) |
| **Chronic left-to-right shunts** |
| ASD <br> VSD <br> PDA <br> Ruptured aortic sinus <br> Aorto-pulmonary window |

**MISTAKES TO AVOID**

- Pulmonary pressures increase with age and weight. So a pulmonary artery systolic pressure of 35–40 mmHg may be a normal finding in an elderly or obese patient.[7]
- IVC size and collapse cannot be used in patients undergoing continuous mechanical ventilation and are unreliable with high positive end expiratory pressures. The pressure from a central line should be used instead.

## CHECKLIST FOR REPORTING IN PULMONARY HYPERTENSION

1. Estimated pulmonary pressures or presence/absence based on time to peak PA velocity and other indirect measures (Table 6.3)
2. RV size and systolic function
3. Tricuspid regurgitation grade
4. Underlying cause

# References

1. Saul T, Lewiss RE, Langsfeld A, Radeos MS, Del Rios M. Inter-rater reliability of sonographic measurements of the inferior vena cava. *J Emerg Med* 2012;42:600–5.
2. Rudski L, Lai W, Afilalo J et al. Guidelines for the echocardiographic assessment of the right heart in adults: a report from the American Society of Echocardiography. *J Am Soc Echocardiogr* 2010;23:685–713.
3. Masuyama T, Kodama K, Kitabatake A et al. Continuous wave Doppler echocardiographic detection of pulmonary regurgitation and its application to noninvasive estimation of pulmonary artery pressure. *Circulation* 1986;74:484–92.
4. Abbas AE, Fortuin FD, Schiller NB et al. Echocardiographic determination of mean pulmonary artery pressure. *Am J Cardiol* 2003;92:1373–6.
5. Kosturakis D, Goldberg SJ, Allen HD, Loeber C. Doppler echocardiographic prediction of pulmonary arterial hypertension in congenital heart disease. *Am J Cardiol* 1984;53:1110–15.
6. McLaughlin VV, Atcher SL, Badesch DB et al. ACCF/AHA 2009 expert consensus document on pulmonary hypertension. *J Am Coll Cardiol* 2009;53:1573–619.
7. McQuillan B, Picard M, Leavitt M, Weyman A. Clinical correlates and reference intervals for pulmonary artery systolic pressure among echocardiographically normal subjects. *Circulation* 2001;104:2797–802.

# Aortic valve disease

## Aortic stenosis

### 1 Appearance of the valve and aorta

- Describe the valve in detail. Look at the number of cusps, pattern of thickening and mobility on zoomed views. These may give a clue to the aetiology (Table 7.1). A bicuspid aortic valve may only be obvious in systole (Figure 7.1).

Table 7.1 Clues to the aetiology in aortic stenosis

|  | Systolic bowing | Closure line | Associated features |
|---|---|---|---|
| Calcific disease | No | Central | Calcification of mitral annulus or aorta |
| Bicuspid | Yes | Eccentric | Ascending aortic dilatation, coarctation |
| Rheumatic | Yes | Central | Mitral involvement |

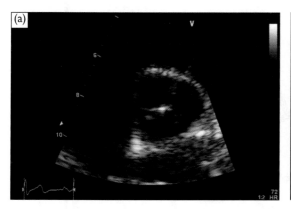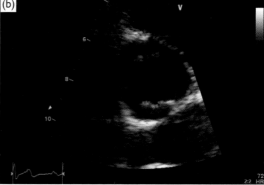

**Figure 7.1 Bicuspid aortic valve in systole and diastole.** In diastole (a) the valve may look tricuspid if there is only mild fusion and no raphe. Only in systole (b) with the valve open will it be obvious that two cusps are partly fused. The fusion may affect only a small length of the cusp edge adjacent to the commissure.

 And here's an electronic link to a loop on the website or use
http://goo.gl/WALt58

- If bicuspid, describe the following:
  - Is it anatomical or functional (two cusps fused either partially or fully with a median raphe)?
  - What is the pattern of fusion? Between right and left cusps is the most common pattern and more likely to be associated with aortic dilatation and coarctation[1] (Figure 7.2).
  - Is the valve thickened and restricted or thin and normally functioning? Thickening and reduced mobility predicts fast progression to surgery.[2]
- Assess the aorta at all levels (see pages 132, 134).
  - In bicuspid aortic valves the sinus, sinotubular junction or ascending aorta may be dilated.
  - If the ascending aorta cannot be imaged adequately even by imaging a space higher than for the parasternal views, consider CMR or CT scanning.
  - The aorta may be replaced at a diameter 45 mm if aortic valve surgery is independently indicated.[8]
  - About 5% of bicuspid valves are associated with coarctation.

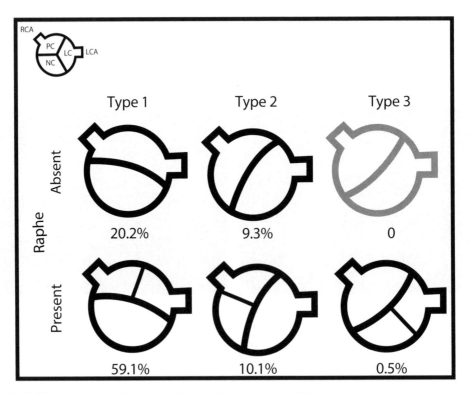

**Figure 7.2 Patterns of fusion.** (Reproduced from The bicuspid aortic valve: an integrated phenotypic classification of leaflet morphology and aortic root shape, Schaefer et al. 94; 1634–8, 2008 with permisssion from BMJ Publishing Group Ltd.)

## 2 Doppler measurements

- The minimum dataset[3] is $V_{max}$, mean gradient and effective orifice area (EOA) using the continuity equation (Appendix 4, section A4.2)
- Record the continuous waveform using the stand-alone probe from the apex and at least one other approach (usually suprasternal or right intercostal) unless the aortic valve disease is obviously mild shown by:
  - mobile cusps and
  - low velocity ($V_{max}$ <3.0 m/s) and
  - normal LV ejection fraction.

## 3 Assess severity

- If the aortic valve is thickened with a $V_{max}$ <2.5 m/s and normal LV ejection fraction, report 'aortic valve thickening with no stenosis'.
- If the $V_{max}$ is ⩾2.5, grade as in Table 7.2 if all measurements agree.[3] If there is disagreement, see 3.1 or 3.2 below.

Table 7.2 Severity in aortic stenosis: main criteria[3]

|  | Mild | Moderate | Severe |
|---|---|---|---|
| Transaortic $V_{max}$ (m/s) | 2.6–2.9 | 3.0–4.0 | >4.0 |
| Peak gradient (mmHg) | <40 | 40–65 | >65 |
| Mean gradient (mmHg) | <20 | 20–40 | >40 |
| EOA (cont eq) (cm²) | >1.5 | 1.0–1.5 | <1.0 |

### 3.1 If the $V_{max}$ suggests severe (>4.0 m/s) but the EOA suggests moderate (>1.0 cm²)

This arises because of:

- high flow (aortic regurgitation, anaemia, anxiety), or
- errors of measurement (pulsed sample too far into the aortic valve or LV diameter too big).

You need to do the following:

- **Check your measurements:** Was the pulsed sample too close to the valve? Check the LV outflow diameter against previous measurements.
- **Consider the dimensionless index** (Table 7.3): If the LV outflow diameter is unreliably large, the dimensionless index gives a guide to severity. It should be calculated as $VTI_{subaortic}/VTI_{ao}$ although the ratio of subaortic to transaortic $V_{max}$ is often used.

- **Look again at the valve appearance:** Is the valve calcified and immobile, suggesting severe aortic stenosis (AS), or are the tips mobile, suggesting more moderate AS?
- **Look at the waveform shape**[3] (Figure 7.3 and Table 7.3): A dagger shape suggests moderate stenosis and an arch shape suggests severe stenosis.
- **Correct for body surface area** (Table 7.3): If the patient is large, a corrected EOA may be in the severe range despite a moderate uncorrected EOA.

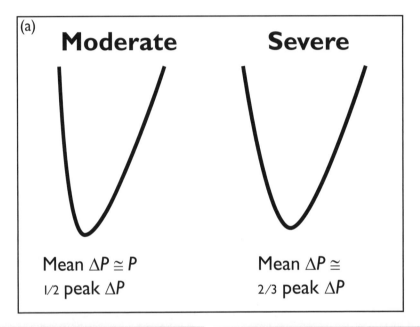

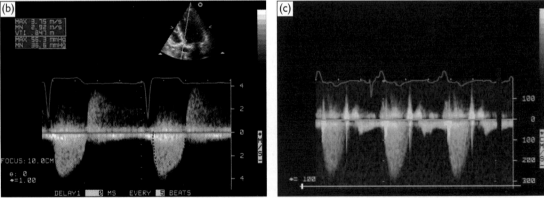

**Figure 7.3 Continuous waveform shape.** (a) Left panel: in moderate aortic stenosis the upstroke is relatively quick, giving a dagger-shaped signal in which the mean gradient is approximately half the peak. Right panel: in severe stenosis the ejection time lengthens and the acceleration time to peak velocity lengthens. This causes an arch shape in which the mean gradient is approximately ⅔ the peak gradient. If the mean to peak ratio is >1.7, the aortic stenosis is moderate; if <1.5, it is severe.[11, 12] (b) A waveform in moderate disease. (c) A waveform in severe disease.

## 3.2 If the $V_{max}$ suggests moderate ($<4.0$ m/s) but the EOA suggests severe ($<1.0$ cm²)

This can be for a number of reasons:

- The cut-points between the grades are to a degree arbitrary and an EOA 0.8–1.0 cm² may be moderate especially in smaller people.[4]
- The EOA is dependent on body size. If the patient is small, a corrected EOA may be in the moderate range despite a 'severe' uncorrected area.
- Low flow causes a fall in $V_{max}$ despite severe aortic stenosis.
- There may be errors of measurement.

Table 7.3 Severity in aortic stenosis: extra criteria

|  | Mild | Moderate | Severe |
|---|---|---|---|
| Waveform shape (Figure 7.3) | Dagger | Dagger | Arch |
| Indexed EOA (cm²/m²) | >0.85 | 0.60–0.85 | <0.60 |
| Dimensionless index | >0.50 | 0.25–0.50 | <0.25 |

You need to do the following:

- **Check your measurements:** The likeliest errors are in placing the pulsed sample too far towards the LV apex and in underestimating LV outflow diameter (check the value found in previous studies).
- **Look again at the valve appearance:** Is the valve calcified and fixed, suggesting severe AS, or are the tips mobile, suggesting moderate AS?
- **Look at the waveform shape[3]** (Figure 7.3 and Table 7.3)**:** A dagger shape suggests moderate stenosis and an arch shape suggests severe.
- **Correct for body surface area if the patient is small.**

## 3.3 Low gradient, low flow aortic stenosis

This occurs if:

- the LV ejection fraction is low; or
- the LV is severely hypertrophied with a small cavity ('paradoxical low flow low gradient AS'). Even with a normal or high ejection fraction the volume of blood ejected is small so that the stroke volume and the systolic flow are both low; or
- there is severe mitral stenosis or regurgitation.

The definition is by a combination of mean gradient <40 mmHg, EOA <1.0 cm² and any one of the following (although only the third measure describes flow directly):

- LV ejection fraction <40%
- stroke volume index <35 ml/m² (see Appendix 4, section A4.4)
- flow <200 ml/s (see Appendix 4, section A4.5)

## 3.4 Consider dobutamine stress echocardiography

- This is indicated if the mean gradient ≤30–40 mmHg and the LV ejection fraction is ≤40%.
- It is not indicated if:
  - the mean gradient >40 mmHg and probably not if >30 mmHg
  - the LV cavity is small and the EF is normal.
- It requires medical supervision because of the risk of cardiac arrhythmia.
  - Give 5 then 10 µg/kg/min dobutamine (occasionally 20 µg/kg/min especially if prior beta-blockade).
  - Stop the infusion if the subaortic velocity integral rises >20% or the heart rate increases.
  - Judge the severity of aortic stenosis and whether there is LV contractile reserve (Table 7.4). If the subaortic velocity integral fails to rise by > 20%, consider calculating the change in flow (see Appendix 4, section A4.5 for calculation).
  - In the absence of contractile reserve, the risk at aortic valve replacement is high.[5]

Table 7.4 Stress echocardiography in low flow aortic stenosis[3]

| Is there severe aortic stenosis? |
| --- |
| Mean gradient >40 mmHg and EOA <1.0 cm² at any time during the infusion |
| Is there LV contractile reserve? |
| Subaortic velocity integral (or ejection fraction or flow) rises by >20% |

## 4 General

- Assess aortic regurgitation (pages 68–71).
- Assess the other valves. Secondary (functional) mitral regurgitation may develop in severe aortic stenosis if the LV is dilated. Mitral surgery is likely to be necessary if:
  - the mitral valve is anatomically abnormal (e.g. prolapsing), or
  - the secondary mitral regurgitation is more than moderate.
- Estimate pulmonary artery pressure. Pulmonary hypertension is common and is a poor prognostic indicator especially in unoperated severe aortic stenosis.[6]
- LV outflow hypertrophy has a number of consequences:
  - It may contribute to high flow velocities across the aortic valve.
  - It may affect a transcatheter aortic valve implantation (TAVI) procedure (see section 6 below).
  - If severe, it increases risk at surgery.

- Postoperatively it contributes to low cardiac output especially with excessive inotropes and diuretic therapy, causing a further decrease in cavity size.

- If there is a discrepancy in the pressure difference and the appearance of the valve, check for a subaortic membrane.

## 5 Is surgery indicated on echocardiography?[7,8]

Aortic valve surgery is most clearly indicated for severe aortic stenosis and symptoms. However, in asymptomatic patients or patients having a coronary artery bypass graft (CABG), the echocardiogram can aid the decision for surgery (Table 7.5).

Table 7.5 Echocardiographic indications for surgery in asymptomatic aortic stenosis[7, 8]

| Indications for surgery |
| --- |
| Moderate or severe AS having CABG or aortic replacement |
| Severe AS and LVEF <50% with no other cause |
| Transaortic $V_{max}$ >5.0 m/s or EOA <0.6 cm² |
| Severe coexistent aortic dilatation (see Table 12.3, pages 134–135) |
| **Less accepted indications*** |
| Increase in $V_{max}$ ≥0.3 m/s in one year associated with severe calcification |
| Severe LV hypertrophy in the absence of systemic hypertension |
| Increase in mean gradient >20 mmHg on exercise |

* These are based on little data (sometimes only one study) and must be interpreted in the whole clinical context

## 6 Transcatheter valve (TAVI) work-up

- Measure the echocardiographic 'annulus' from inner to inner edge at the base of the cusps.[9] This is needed for sizing the valve.
- The annulus may be oval. Further assessment of the annulus size and shape may be performed at the TAVI centre using:
  - 3D TOE performed at the time of the procedure or beforehand if there is significant uncertainty[10]
  - CT.

Features of the work-up are summarised in Table 7.6.

Table 7.6 Echocardiographic features in the TAVI work-up

| Aorta | |
| --- | --- |
| Heavy calcification | Confirms TAVI more suitable than conventional surgery |
| Annulus diameter | Used for sizing |
| Diameter at sinus and STJ | Dilatation (>45 mm) may contraindicate Corevalve |
| **Left ventricle** | |
| LV cavity size | If small, contraindicates transapical approach |
| Severe subaortic bulge | May contraindicate SAPIEN |
| **Valves** | |
| Bicuspid valve | Caution with some types of device |
| Heavy calcification L cusp | Caution re occlusion of left main stem (LMS) during the procedure |
| Severe MR | May favour conventional surgery |

## 7 Other techniques

- **CT** is useful:
  - to detect dilatation and tortuosity of the ascending aorta if this is not imaged adequately on echo
  - if porcelain aorta is suspected from the echo or the coronary angiogram
  - in the work-up towards TAVI to assess:
    - the annulus (area, perimeter, diameters, shape and calcification)
    - the height of the coronary ostia above the annulus
  - to assess the whole thoracic aorta
  - gives a calcium score which may aid the differentiation of moderate and severe AS
  - can assess coronary anatomy preoperatively.
- **CMR** is useful:
  - to detect dilatation of the ascending aorta if this is not imaged adequately on echocardiography
  - to image subaortic obstruction (midcavity muscular obstruction, subaortic membranes) if not imaged adequately on echocardiography.

 **MISTAKES TO AVOID**

- Mistaking the continuous wave signal from an eccentric jet of mitral regurgitation for aortic stenosis

- Failing to recognise severe aortic stenosis if the $V_{max}$ or mean gradient is in the moderate range but the EOA is low
- Underestimating the degree of aortic stenosis by not using a stand-alone probe from at least two windows
- Failing to detect dilatation of the ascending aorta, which is common if there is a bicuspid aortic valve
- Missing a subaortic membrane. Consider if the valve looks relatively mildly affected but the velocities are high

## CHECKLIST FOR REPORTING AORTIC STENOSIS

1. Appearance and movement of the aortic valve
2. Grade of stenosis
3. Grade of associated regurgitation
4. Size of aorta and check for coarctation
5. Left ventricular dimensions and systolic function
6. Other valves
7. Pulmonary artery pressure

# Aortic regurgitation

## 1 Appearance of the valve and aorta

- Describe the valve in detail. Look at the number of cusps and mobility on zoomed views. (See Figure 7.1 for bicuspid aortic valve.)
- Measure the aorta at every standard level (see pages 132 and 134).
- This may allow you to determine the aetiology (Table 7.7).

Table 7.7  Aetiology of aortic regurgitation

| Dilatation of root or ascending aorta | |
|---|---|
| See Table 12.1 | |
| **Valve** | |
| Common | Bicuspid, rheumatic, calcific disease, endocarditis |
| Uncommon | Prolapse, irradiation, drugs (cabergoline, pergolide, fenfluramine, benfluorex, ecstasy), antiphospholipid syndrome, carcinoid |

## 2 Colour flow mapping

- Measure the jet height 5–10 mm below the cusps (on 2D or colour M-mode) (Figure 7.4) and express as a percentage of the diameter of the LV outflow tract (LVOT).
- If the jet is eccentric, the width must be taken perpendicular to its axis. If it is so eccentric that it impinges on the septum or anterior mitral leaflet, the method is unreliable.
- The width of the narrowest portion of the jet (the vena contracta) can also be used (Table 7.8).

## 3 Continuous wave signal

- Record either from the apex or, if the jet is directed posteriorly, from the parasternal position
- Measure the pressure half-time and note the density of the signal compared with the density of forward flow.

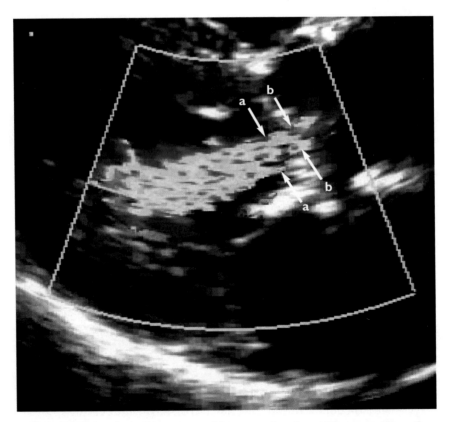

**Figure 7.4 Regurgitant jet.** Parasternal long-axis view. The position for measuring the height of the colour flow map as a percentage of the outflow tract height is at a. The vena contracta or neck is at b.

## 4 Flow reversal at the arch

From the suprasternal notch describe:

● whether flow reversal is holodiastolic, fills approximately half of diastole or is only seen at the start of diastole using colour M-mode (Figure 7.5) and pulsed Doppler (Figure 7.6)

● how far down the aorta can flow reversal be detected on colour mapping.

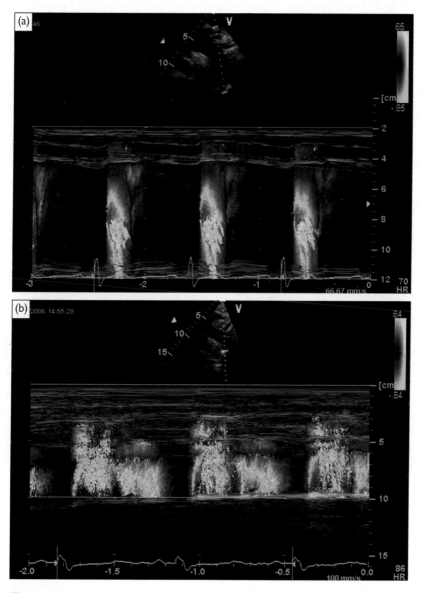

**Figure 7.5 Flow reversal on colour mapping in the upper descending thoracic aorta.** Using a suprasternal position, colour M-mode in a patient with mild regurgitation (a) illustrates localised and short-lived flow reversal. In severe regurgitation (b) flow reversal is holodiastolic across the whole aortic lumen and seen well down the descending thoracic aorta.

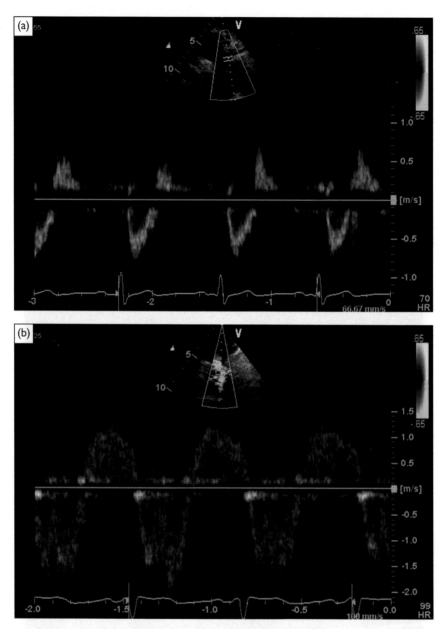

**Figure 7.6 Flow reversal on pulsed Doppler in the distal arch.** Using a suprasternal position. Mild regurgitation causes short-lived low velocity reversal (a), while in severe regurgitation the reversal is holodiastolic with a relatively high velocity at the end of diastole (e.g. ≥0.2 m/s) (b).[18]

# 5 Grade the severity of regurgitation

- Make an assessment based on all modalities. The height of the colour jet in the LV outflow tract and flow reversal beyond the arch are the most reliable modalities (Table 7.8).

Table 7.8 Criteria of severity in aortic regurgitation[13, 14]

|  | Mild | Moderate | Severe |
|---|---|---|---|
| Colour /LVOT height (%) | <25 | 25–64 | ≥65 |
| Vena contracta width (mm) | <3 | 3–6 | >6 |
| Flow reversal indescending aorta | None | Not holodiastolic | Holodiastolic |
| Pressure half-time (ms) | >500 | 200–500 | <200*† |
| CW signal intensity | Faint or incomplete waveform | Intermediate | Dense as forward flow |

*A cut-off of 200 ms appears in both ASE and European guidelines, but a number of individual studies[15] suggest a threshold of <300 ms

†The pressure half-time depends on LV diastolic pressure and systemic vascular resistance and may be short with LV dysfunction even if the aortic regurgitation is mild or moderate

- Also take into account the size and activity of the left ventricle.
- The PISA technique is not routinely used for aortic regurgitation.

## 6 The left ventricle

- Is the LV hyperdynamic (suggesting severe aortic regurgitation)? Chronic severe regurgitation usually causes LV diastolic dilatation. In acute regurgitation the LV diastolic volume may be normal.
- Measure LV volumes because the LV becomes more spherical in severe aortic regurgitation and linear dimensions may then be unreliable for serial echocardiography. No firm cut-point for surgery exists but one study[16] suggests an LV systolic volume ≥45 ml/m$^2$. A progressive change is more useful than a single cut-point.
- Tissue Doppler systolic velocity can corroborate a decline in other measures of LV function but cannot be used on its own as an indication for surgery in the absence of sufficient data. In one study a tissue Doppler systolic velocity <9.5 cm/s measured at the medial mitral annulus was an indicator of poor exercise response.[17]
- In acute aortic regurgitation, a transmitral E deceleration time <150 ms indicates high filling pressures with a high risk of decompensation.

## 7 Are there echocardiographic criteria for surgery?[7, 8]

In asymptomatic severe aortic regurgitation, indications for surgery are:
- an LV systolic diameter >50 mm (or 25 mm/m$^2$)
- an LV diastolic diameter >70 mm[8] (>65[7]), i.e. the threshold is different between AHA and ESC guidelines

- LV ejection fraction ≤50%
- aortic dilatation (see Table 12.3, pages 134–135)
- a combination of changes in LV and aortic dimensions and the grade of regurgitation outside these cut-points in individual cases.

## 8 Assess the other valves and right heart

- Functional mitral regurgitation may occur secondary to LV dilatation.
- Pulmonary hypertension is much less common than in severe aortic stenosis.

## 9 Other techniques

- **CMR:**
  - shows valve morphology if echocardiographic windows are suboptimal
  - shows the rest of the aorta if only the root can be imaged adequately on echocardiography
  - estimates the regurgitant fraction if the grade of regurgitation is uncertain on echocardiography
  - calculates LV volume and function if image quality is suboptimal on echocardiography.
- **CT:**
  - shows valve morphology if echocardiographic windows are suboptimal
  - shows the rest of the aorta if only the root can be imaged adequately on echocardiography
  - can assess coronary anatomy preoperatively.

 **MISTAKES TO AVOID**

- Placing the pulsed sample in the distal arch too close to the aortic wall. This produces signal artefacts late in diastole (signal symmetrical above and below the baseline) which can be mistaken for flow reversal (flow above the baseline only)
- Missing a transmitral deceleration time <150 ms as a sign of imminent decompensation in acute aortic regurgitation
- Overestimating AR using AR pressure half-time shortened by a high left ventricular end-diastolic pressure (LVEDP) as a result of coexistent LV disease
- Using vena contracta cut-points to assess the jet width in the LV outflow tract
- Measuring pressure half-time when not fully aligned to the regurgitant jet. The AR jet initial peak velocity should be about 4 m/s; if much lower, especially with a bidirectional signal, use other methods to evaluate the degree of regurgitation

## CHECKLIST FOR REPORTING AORTIC REGURGITATION

1. Appearance of aortic valve
2. Grade of regurgitation
3. Aortic dimensions
4. LV dimensions and systolic function
5. Mitral valve

## References

1. Schaefer BM, Lewin MB, Stout KK et al. The bicuspid aortic valve: an integrated phenotypic classification of leaflet morphology and aortic root shape. *Heart* 2008;94:1634–8.
2. Michelena HI, Desjardins VA, Avierinos JF et al. Natural history of asymptomatic patients with normally functioning or minimally dysfunctional bicuspid aortic valve in the community. *Circulation* 2008;117:2776–84.
3. Baumgartner H, Hung J, Bermejo J et al. Echocardiographic assessment of valve stenosis: EAE/ASE recommendations for clinical practice. *Eur J Echocardiogr* 2009;10:1–25.
4. Minners J, Allgeir M, Gohlke-Baerwolf C, Kienzle RP, Neuman FJ, Jander N. Inconsistencies of echocardiographic criteria for the grading of aortic stenosis. *Eur Heart J* 2008;29:1043–8.
5. Monin J-L, Quere J-P, Moncho M et al. Low-gradient aortic stenosis. Operative risk stratification and predictors for long-term outcome: a multicenter study using dobutamine stress hemodynamics. *Circulation* 2003;108:319–24.
6. Cam A, Goel SS, Agarwal S et al. Prognostic implications of pulmonary hypertension in patients with severe aortic stenosis. *J Thorac Cardiovasc Surg* 2011;142:80–8.
7. Nishimura RA, Otto CM, Bonow RO et al. 2014 AHA/ACC guideline for the management of patients with valvular heart disease. *J Am Coll Cardiol* 2014;63:e57–e185.
8. Vahanian A, Alfieri O, Andreotti F et al. Guidelines on the management of valvular heart disease (version 2012). *Eur Heart J* 2012;33:2451–96.
9. Zamorano JL, Badano LP, Bruce C et al. EAE/ASE recommendations for the use of echocardiography in new transcatheter interventions for valvular heart disease. *Eur Heart J* 2011;32(17):2189–214.
10. Rajani R, Hancock J, Chambers J. Imaging: the art of TAVI. *Heart* 2012;98 (Suppl 4): iv14–iv22.
11. Chambers J, Rajani R, Hankins M, Cook R. The peak to mean pressure drop ratio: a new method of assessing aortic stenosis. *J Am Soc Echocardiogr* 2005;18:674–8.
12. Haghi D, Kaden JJ, Suselbeck T et al. Validation of the peak to mean pressure decrease ratio as a new method of assessing aortic stenosis using the Gorlin formula and the cardiovascular magnetic resonance-based hybrid method. *Echocardiography* 2007;24:335–9.

13. Lancellotti P, Tribouilloy C, Hagendorff A et al. European Association of Echocardiography recommendations for the assessment of valvular regurgitation. Part 1: aortic and pulmonary regurgitation (native valve disease). *Eur J Echocardiogr* 2010;11:223–44.

14. Zoghbi WA, Enriquez-Sarano M, Foster E et al. Recommendations for evaluation of the severity of native valvular regurgitation with two-dimensional and Doppler echocardiography. *J Am Soc Echocardiogr* 2003;16(7):777–802.

15. Teague SM, Heinsimer JA, Anderson JL et al. Quantification of aortic regurgitation utilizing continuous wave Doppler ultrasound. *J Am Coll Cardiol* 1986;8(3):592–9.

16. Detaint D, Messika-Zeitoun D, Maalouf J et al. Quantitative echocardiographic determinants of clinical outcome in asymptomatic patients with aortic regurgitation: a prospective study. *J Am Coll Cardiol Imaging* 2008;1(1):1–11.

17. Vinereanu D, Ionescu AA, Fraser AG. Assessment of LV long-axis contraction can detect early myocardial dysfunction in asymptomatic patients with severe AR. *Heart* 2001;85:30–6.

18. Tribouilloy C, Avinee P, Shen WF, Rey JL, Slama M, Lesbre JP. End diastolic flow velocity just beneath the aortic isthmus assessed by pulsed Doppler echocardiography: a new predictor of the aortic regurgitant fraction. *Br Heart J* 1991;65(1):37–40.

# Mitral valve disease

8

## Mitral stenosis

### 1 Appearance of the valve, annulus and chordae

- Almost all mitral stenosis is rheumatic in origin (Table 8.1). Rheumatic disease is shown by:
  - commissural fusion (seen in the PS short-axis)
  - bowing of the tips
  - thickening of the leaflet tips
  - chordal thickening.
- Degenerative calcification in the annulus is increasingly common but usually causes no more than moderate stenosis. It may be hard to image the relatively thin and mobile leaflets.

Table 8.1 Causes of mitral stenosis

| Common |
| --- |
| Rheumatic disease |
| Calcific annular disease |
| **Uncommon** |
| Radiation |
| Systemic lupus erythematosus |
| Congenital |

### 2 Planimeter the orifice area

- Make sure that the section is not oblique. This is aided by 3D (Figure 8.1).
- Use colour Doppler as a guide to the extent of the orifice if this is not obvious on imaging.
- Take care not to include the chordae which, if thickened, can mimic the orifice.
- If there is significant thickening with reverberation artefact, the measurement may be inaccurate and should not be made.
- In calcific annular disease, planimetry may not be feasible. If colour fills the orifice in all views with no major aliasing and a width >10 mm, there is no significant stenosis.

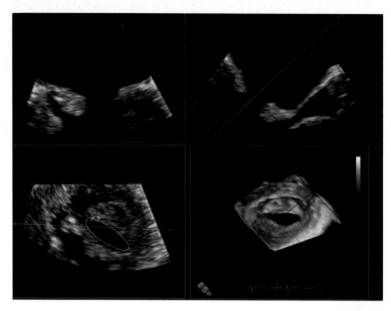

**Figure 8.1 Planimetry of the mitral orifice.** The orifice is imaged in a parasternal short-axis view. Care must be taken to section the tips of the mitral leaflets perpendicularly. A common mistake is to section towards the base of the leaflets or across thickened chordae.

Table 8.2 Criteria of severity in mitral stenosis[1]

|  | Mild | Moderate | Severe |
|---|---|---|---|
| Orifice area by planimetry (cm²) | >1.5 | 1.0–1.5 | <1.0 |
| Pressure half-time (ms) | <150 | 150–220 | >220 |
| Mean gradient (mmHg) | <5 | 5–10 | >10* |
| PA pressure (mmHg) | <30 | 30–50 | >50† |

*>15 mmHg after exercise

†The relationship with grade of valve stenosis is not tight

## 3 Continuous wave signal

- Average the pressure half-time and mean gradient over 3–5 cycles if there is atrial fibrillation.
- The Hatle formula (orifice area = 220/pressure half-time) is an approximate guide to severity in moderate or severe stenosis.
- In calcific annular disease there is often a large transmitral A wave as a result of long-standing systemic hypertension (Figure 8.2). This can lead to overestimation of the severity of mitral stenosis using the threshold mean gradients derived from patients in atrial fibrillation with no A wave. Usually the leaflet tips will be imaged as thin and mobile and the size of the orifice on colour-mapping can be the primary measure of severity.

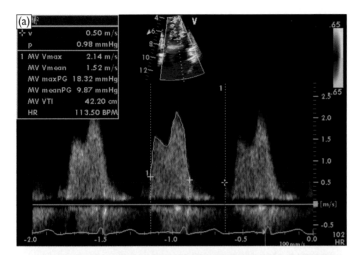

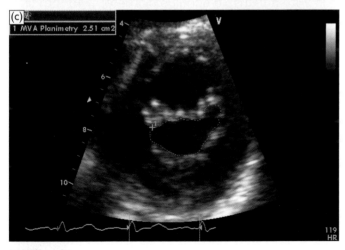

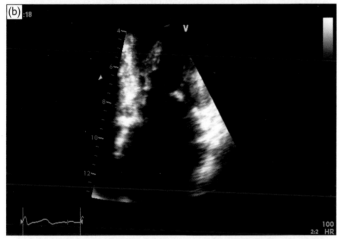

Figure 8.2 Pseudosevere mitral stenosis. In patients with a calcified mitral annulus, it is uncommon for the stenosis to be severe. However, there may be a large A wave as a result of underlying LV diastolic dysfunction. This can increase the estimated transmitral gradient to levels suggesting severe stenosis despite a moderate orifice area. In this example the mean gradient is 9 mmHg (a) despite a mobile valve (b) with an orifice area of 2.5 cm² (c).

And here's an electronic link to a loop on the website or use
http://goo.gl/EDsYfs

## 4 Assess mitral regurgitation

See pages 84–87.

- Anything more than mild mitral regurgitation means that the valve is not suitable for valvotomy.
- The transmitral pressure half-time will be shortened disproportionate to the orifice area if there is severe mitral (or aortic) regurgitation.
- Mean transmitral gradient will increase with significant mitral regurgitation.

## 5 Assess severity of mitral stenosis

See Table 8.2 (page 76).

- The planimetered orifice area is the most reliable measure in rheumatic disease if performed accurately. The gradient and pulmonary artery pressure are flow-dependent.

## 6 Examine the right heart

- The pulmonary artery pressure (see Chapter 6) has a loose relationship with the severity of mitral stenosis, and pulmonary hypertension is a criterion for balloon valvotomy:[2]
  - pulmonary artery systolic pressure >50 mmHg at rest.
- Right ventricular dilatation with hypokinesis is a more important predictor of poor outcome at mitral valve surgery than the pulmonary artery pressure which may fall after mitral valve replacement.
- Tricuspid rheumatic involvement is common, but easily missed.
- Mild or more tricuspid regurgitation with a tricuspid annulus diameter ⩾40 mm (in diastole on a 4-chamber view) (>21 mm/m[2]) is currently an indication for tricuspid annuloplasty at the time of mitral valve replacement[3, 4] in rheumatic disease but based on few data.

## 7 Assess the other valves

- Significant aortic valve disease may mean that double valve replacement rather than balloon mitral valvotomy is indicated.
- Aortic stenosis can be underestimated because of low flow caused by severe mitral stenosis (or regurgitation).
- The transmitral pressure half-time will be shortened disproportionate to the orifice area if there is severe aortic regurgitation.

## 8 Risk of atrial thrombus

- Transthoracic echocardiography is insensitive for detecting thrombus. A transoesophageal study should always be performed before balloon valvotomy.

- A dilated left atrium is a criterion for considering warfarin in severe mitral stenosis and sinus rhythm:[2, 5]
  - diameter on M-mode >50 mm, or
  - volume >60 ml/m$^2$.

## 9 Is the valve suitable for balloon valvotomy?

- The most reliable characteristics of the valve for predicting success without developing severe mitral regurgitation are given in Table 8.3.[6]

Table 8.3 Markers of successful balloon valvotomy

| |
| --- |
| Good mobility of the anterior leaflet |
| No more than minor chordal involvement |
| No more than mild mitral regurgitation |
| No commissural calcification |
| No left atrial thrombus (on TOE) |

Some centres use the Wilkins system of scoring 1 to 4 for valve mobility, thickening calcification and subvalvar involvement[7] (Appendix 3, Table A3.2, page 220) with a score ≤8 suggesting that balloon valvotomy will be successful. However, this system does not focus on the important markers (Table 8.3).

 **MISTAKES TO AVOID**

- Off-axis planimetry of the mitral valve
- Failing to take account of the effects of severe MR or AR on transmitral pressure half-time
- Overestimating the degree of stenosis in patients with a heavily calcified annulus in sinus rhythm because of a large A wave

**CHECKLIST FOR REPORTING MITRAL STENOSIS**

1. Appearance of valve
2. Severity of stenosis and regurgitation
3. Right-sided pressures and right ventricular function
4. Other valves
5. Is the valve suitable for balloon valvotomy?

# Mitral regurgitation

## 1 Appearance and movement of the valve

- Mitral regurgitation is either primary (caused by an abnormality of the valve) or secondary (caused by an abnormality of the ventricle) (Table 8.4). In primary MR the valve looks abnormal while in secondary MR the valve looks normal but is restricted ('tented') in systole (Table 8.4).
- The mitral valve apparatus consists of the leaflets, chordae, annulus and adjacent myocardium. However, the main clues to the aetiology are in the leaflets themselves.

**Table 8.4** Causes of mitral regurgitation

| Cause | Valve appearance | Movement | Jet direction |
|---|---|---|---|
| **Primary (organic), i.e. abnormal mitral valve** | | | |
| Floppy mitral valve | Variable myxomatous change | Prolapse in systole | Away from prolapse |
| Rheumatic disease | Thickened tips | Bowing in diastole | Usually central |
| Endocarditis | Vegetation, destruction | Sections of valve may move out of phase | Variable |
| Other: SLE, drugs | Generalised thickening | Systolic restriction | Usually central |
| **Secondary (functional), i.e. abnormal LV\*** | | | |
| Inferoposterior infarct | Normal | Posterior restriction | Posterior |
| Inf and ant infarct | Normal | Symmetrical restriction | Central |
| Global LV dilatation | Normal | Usually symmetrical restriction | Central |

\*Papillary muscle rupture is usually considered separately as acute ischaemic mitral regurgitation. 'Ischaemic mitral regurgitation' is used for secondary mitral regurgitation caused by myocardial infarction

### 1.1 Appearance of the valve

- Thickened leaflet tips are typical of rheumatic disease often with rigid posterior leaflet, commissural fusion, and chordal thickening and matting.
- Generalised thickening occurs in antiphospholipid syndrome or late after high-dose radiation or after drugs (cabergoline, pergolide, phentermine, ecstasy).

- A floppy valve may only look thickened as prolapse develops in systole and is often associated with lax chordae and a dilated mitral annulus.
- A discrete mass attached to the leaflet suggests a vegetation (page 125).
  - In the context of an acute coronary syndrome, consider a ruptured papillary muscle tip.
  - A ruptured chord is usually a thin whip-like structure associated with prolapse.

## 1.2 Movement

- Is there evidence of prolapse (Table 8.5, page 82 and Figure 8.3, page 81)?
  - Does it affect anterior or posterior leaflets or both?
  - Which segments are involved using the Carpentier classification (Figure 8.4)?
  - Does prolapse affect the leaflet tip, the whole leaflet (like a bucket handle) or is it flail (moving through 180° and often with a visible ruptured chord)?

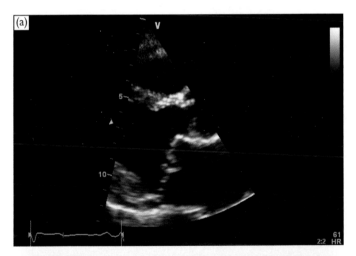

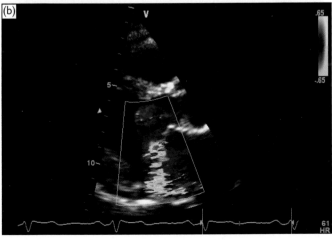

**Figure 8.3 Mitral prolapse.** In this image, the anterior leaflet prolapses (a) and the regurgitant jet is directed posteriorly (b), away from the abnormal leaflet.

81

**Table 8.5** Signs of mitral prolapse

| |
|---|
| Movement of part of either leaflet >2 mm behind the plane of the annulus in the parasternal or apical long-axis views |
| Displacement of the point of coaption behind the plane of the annulus in the 4-chamber view. |
| Prolapse of A3, P3 or the medial commissure may be seen in the apical 2-chamber view, parasternal short-axis view or the parasternal long-axis view tilted towards the right ventricle |
| Prolapse of A1, P1 or the lateral commissure may be seen in the apical 2-chamber view, parasternal short-axis view or the parasternal long-axis view tilted towards the pulmonary artery |

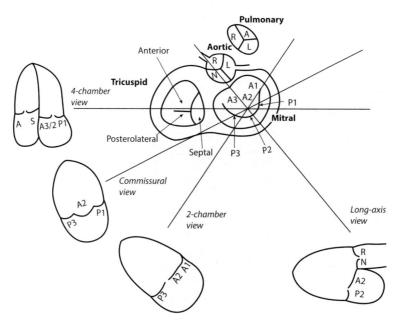

**Figure 8.4 Mitral valve segments according to the Carpentier classification on transthoracic examination.** This scheme includes a view through the commissures adapted from transoesophageal echocardiography. This can often be obtained transthoracically by slight angulation and rotation from the apical 2-chamber view.

- Is there restriction of opening in diastole?
  - Restriction of both leaflet tips alone with bowing of the leaflets occurs in rheumatic disease.
  - Confusion occasionally arises because of reduced opening of the whole of both leaflets (not just the tip) as a result of low cardiac output or of the anterior leaflet alone because of an impinging jet of aortic regurgitation.
- Is there restriction of both leaflets during systole (symmetrical tenting) (Figure 8.5 and Table 8.6)?

- This is usually associated with severe LV systolic dysfunction, either a globally dilated and hypokinetic LV or myocardial infarction in both inferior and anterior territories.
- The MR jet is directed centrally.

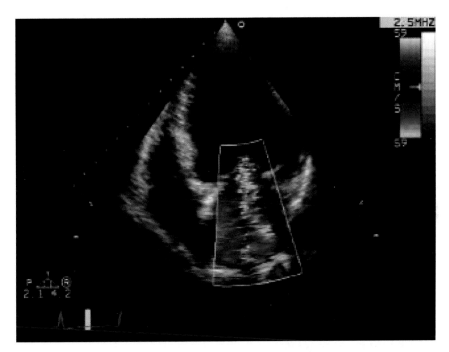

**Figure 8.5 Functional mitral regurgitation.** In functional regurgitation, as a result of symmetrical tenting of the leaflets, the regurgitant jet is central; if one leaflet is slightly more restricted than the other, the jet will be directed towards that leaflet.

Table 8.6 Restricted leaflet motion

| **Both leaflets** |
| --- |
| Tenting (point of apposition above the plane of the annulus in the 4-chamber view) |
| Centrally directed jet of regurgitation (Figure 8.5) |
| Dilated left ventricle causing abnormal papillary muscle function |
| **Restriction of posterior leaflet motion** |
| Tip of leaflet held in left ventricle during systole (best seen in a long-axis view) (Figure 3.1) |
| Jet directed posteriorly (Figure 3.1, page 23) |
| Inferior or posterior infarct |

- Is there restriction of the posterior leaflet during systole (asymmetrical tenting) (see Figure 3.1, page 23)?
  - This is usually associated with an inferior or posterior infarction which may be small. Occasionally it is caused by fibrotic shortening of the chordate.
  - The restriction may be subtle.
  - The MR jet is directed posteriorly.
- If the leaflets look normal and move normally:
  - Check the annulus diameter. A diameter >35 mm in women and >40 mm in men raises the suspicion of dilatation[8] (Appendix 3, Table A3.1). Isolated annulus dilatation can cause severe MR even without leaflet prolapse or LV dysfunction.
  - Check for a perforation or cleft.
  - Check for commissural prolapse:
    - The jet origin will be to the medial or lateral part of the orifice in the PS short-axis view.
    - A jet from the commissure imaged in the PS LA view may be mistaken for a perforation.
    - Angling from the PS long-axis view medially towards the RV or laterally towards the PA will bring the prolapse into view.
  - The abnormality may be more obvious on 3D. If image quality is suboptimal, consider TOE.

## 2 Colour flow mapping

The following should be assessed:
- The origin of the jet (e.g. medial, central or lateral part of the orifice).
- The direction of the jet:
  - away from a prolapsing leaflet (Figure 8.3b)
  - behind a restricted leaflet (Figure 3.1b)
  - centrally if symmetrical 'tenting' of the leaflets (Figure 8.5) or usually in rheumatic disease.
- The width of the jet at the level of the orifice using either:
  - the vena contracta width averaged from all views in which it is seen well (Figure 8.6), or
  - the PISA method (Figure 8.7).
- The size of the flow convergence zone within the left ventricle is assessed by eye.
- The duration of the jet using colour M-mode:
  - Is it holosystolic or present only in part of systole (usually the latter part as prolapse develops in bileaflet prolapse)?
  - The quantification of a jet based on jet width or PISA has to be modified by an arbitrary factor if is non holosystolic.

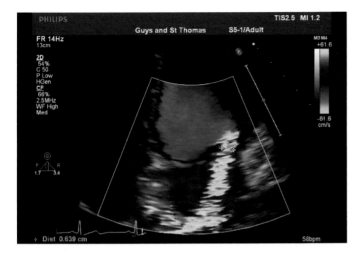

**Figure 8.6 Vena contracta.** An average diameter should be given from orthogonal views to take account of the cross-section on the jet being oval rather than circular.

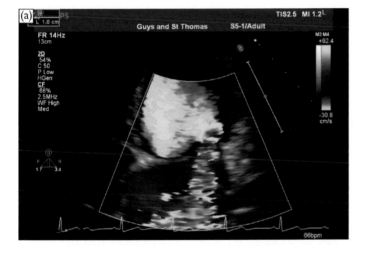

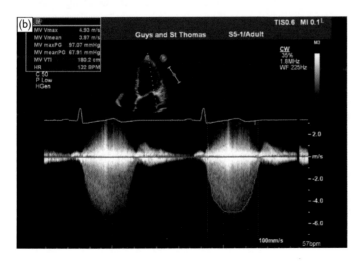

**Figure 8.7 The PISA method.**

- Lower the image depth to increase the size of the area of interest.
- Reduce the Nyquist limit to 15–40 cm/s.
- Measure the radius ($r$ in cm) of the first aliasing shell at mid-systole. $V_a$ in cm/s is the Nyquist limit.
- Measure the peak velocity ($V_{cw}$ in m/s) and velocity time integral ($VTI_{cw}$ in cm) of the continuous wave mitral regurgitant signal (Figure 8.7b).
- The formulae are:
  - EROA (in mm²) = $(2\pi r^2 V_a / V_{cw})$
  - R vol (in ml) = (EROA × $VTI_{cw}$)/100 (in ml)

85

## 3 Continuous wave signal

- Look at the shape and density of the signal. A signal as dense as forward flow suggests severe regurgitation, a low intensity or incomplete signal mild regurgitation and an intermediate signal moderate regurgitation
- Rapid depressurisation of the signal causes a 'dagger-shaped' signal and is a sign of severe regurgitation.

## 4 Pulsed Doppler

- Severe mitral regurgitation is suggested by:
  - a high transmitral E wave velocity (>1.5 m/s) in the absence of mitral stenosis
  - the ratio of transmitral velocity integral to subaortic velocity integral[9] >1.4.
- A pulsed sample in a pulmonary vein at a distance from the jet can aid quantification although this is most useful TOE. Blunting of the systolic signal occurs in moderate and severe regurgitation; flow reversal in very severe regurgitation.
- The estimation of filling pressures using the E/E' ratio (transmitral E wave velocity/ Doppler tissue systolic velocity) is not valid in the presence of severe mitral regurgitation.

## 5 Left ventricular function

- Measure linear dimensions at the base of the heart. The systolic dimension is particularly important and should be averaged over several measurements. In regurgitation caused by a floppy valve, surgery can be considered even in the absence of symptoms if the systolic dimension is 40 mm and the valve is repairable at low risk.[2, 10]
- Left ventricular shape may often change in severe mitral regurgitation and LV systolic volume (biplane Simpson's method or 3D) aids the detection of progressive LV dilatation on serial studies.

## 6 General

### 6.1 Assess the left atrium

- A dilated left atrium is a non-specific sign of chronic severe regurgitation (but also occurs in atrial fibrillation, systemic hypertension, etc.).
- Progressive LA dilatation is a minor indication for surgery in asymptomatic patients with repairable mitral valves.[2] The current suggested threshold is $\geq$60 ml/m$^2$.

### 6.2 Assess the right heart

- Pulmonary hypertension may complicate severe mitral regurgitation.

- A PA pressure >50 mmHg at rest is an indication for surgery in asymptomatic severe mitral regurgitation if the valve is repairable.[2]

## 6.3 Assess the other valves

- The significance of aortic stenosis may be underestimated from the transaortic velocities as a result of low forward flow in severe mitral regurgitation.
- Tricuspid annuloplasty may be considered at the time of mitral valve surgery if there is moderate or worse tricuspid regurgitation and a tricuspid annulus diameter ≥40 mm measured in diastole in a 4-chamber view.

# 7 Grading regurgitation

Table 8.7 Grading mitral regurgitation[9, 11]*

|  | Mild | Moderate* | | Severe |
|---|---|---|---|---|
| Neck width (mm) | <3 | 3–6.9 | | ≥7 |
| Flow convergence zone | Absent | Moderate | | Large |

| **PISA quantities** | | | | |
|---|---|---|---|---|
|  | Mild | Mild-moderate | Moderate-severe | Severe |
| EROA (mm²)† | <20 | 20–29 | 30–39 | ≥40 |
| Regurgitant volume (ml) | <30 | 30–44 | 45–59 | ≥60 |
| RF (%) | <30 | 30–39 | 40–49 | ≥50 |

*This table uses data from the EAE and ASE publications.[9, 11] Subsequent guidelines[2] on the management of valve disease made the threshold for severe secondary MR the same as for moderate primary MR because the risk of events rises at lower grades for secondary than for primary regurgitation.[12] Furthermore, the PISA method is less representative in secondary MR where the jet may be oval rather than circular in cross section (this is less of a problem using an averaged vena contracta width). We suggest that having different thresholds for primary and secondary MR is confusing and not necessary. The clinician in charge of the case should be relied upon to interpret reported moderate regurgitation as clinically appropriate

†EROA: Effective regurgitant orifice area using PISA method

Make a judgement based on all modalities with the specific signs in Table 8.7 supported by:

- density and shape of the continuous wave signal
- a hyperdynamic LV
- pulmonary hypertension.

**MISTAKES TO AVOID**

- Confusion about the different cut-points for severe in secondary compared with primary mitral regurgitation.[2, 12] We suggest using the same assessment methods, as described above, for all types of MR but being aware that invasive intervention may be indicated for moderate secondary mitral regurgitation
- A hyperdynamic LV suggests severe MR so think twice before reporting mild or moderate MR
- Missing early LV dysfunction because LVEF is in the low normal range for a left ventricle with normal loading (see Table 2.6)
- Not looking for MR after myocardial infarction or in aortic valve disease when it affects therapy
- Mistaking posterior restriction for anterior prolapse (both cause a posteriorly directed jet of regurgitation)
- Excessive use of TOE when the information needed is obtainable on transthoracic echocardiography (TTE)

## CHECKLIST FOR REPORTING MITRAL REGURGITATION

1. Detailed description of the valve appearance and movement including mechanism (and, if possible, cause)
2. Severity of regurgitation
3. Left ventricular dimensions, volume and systolic function
4. The right heart including:
   a. pulmonary artery pressure
   b. tricuspid annulus diameter
5. Left atrial size
6. Presence of other valve disease

# Specialist pre- and postoperative assessment

## 1 Surgery in primary (organic) mitral regurgitation

- In asymptomatic patients with severe primary MR the indications for surgery (Table 8.8) depend on LV systolic size and the likelihood of repair (Table 8.9) as well as non-echocardiographic features (e.g. comorbidities and patient choice).

- Isolated P2 prolapse is easily amenable to repair. More complex prolapse may be less easy to repair. Repair is not usually possible or attempted for:
  - rheumatic disease, except in countries where adequate anticoagulation control for a mechanical replacement valve is not feasible
  - extensive mitral valve thickening and prolapse
  - extensive destruction especially in acute endocarditis
  - extensive annular calcification.

**Table 8.8** Indications for surgery in asymptomatic patients with primary mitral regurgitation[2, 10]

| If repair is not certain |
|---|
| LVSD $\geqslant$45 mm ($\geqslant$40 mm*) or EF $\leqslant$60% |
| PA systolic pressure at rest >50 mmHg |
| **If there is a high likelihood of repair** |
| LVSD $\geqslant$40 mm (or <40 mm if repair near certain at a 'valve center of excellence'*) |
| †LA volume $\geqslant$60 ml/m² |
| †PA systolic pressure on exercise $\geqslant$60 mmHg |

†Class IIb indications, i.e. not universally accepted
*Nishimura et al, 2014

- If the tricuspid annulus is >40 mm (>21 mm/m²) and there is moderate or severe tricuspid regurgitation (associated with mitral prolapse) or mild or more tricuspid regurgitation (associated with rheumatic disease), it is recommended to perform tricuspid annuloplasty at the time of mitral valve surgery.

## 2 Surgery in secondary (functional) mitral regurgitation

There are some differences from primary mitral regurgitation.

- The prognostic significance of moderate secondary regurgitation is similar to that of more severe primary regurgitation.[12]
- Indications for mitral surgery (Table 8.9) depend on LV function, the presence of myocardial viability and the absence of adverse factors (Figure 8.8) of which the most important are:
  - broad and eccentric jet
  - small or normal mitral annulus (<35 mm as a guide)
  - severe tenting (tenting height >10 mm or area $\geqslant$2.5 cm²).
- There is a greater role for stress echocardiography. Patients with leaflet tenting and ischaemic disease are more likely to increase the degree of mitral regurgitation on exercise.

- Exercise echocardiography is indicated for:
  - patients with breathlessness out of proportion to the grade of MR or LV dysfunction
  - patients with mild or moderate MR about to have CABG
  - acute pulmonary oedema without cause.
- Dobutamine stress echocardiography is indicated for patients with an impaired LV to determine whether there is evidence of viability.

Table 8.9 Indications for surgery in secondary mitral regurgitation[2, 10]

| Having CABG anyway |
| --- |
| Moderate or severe MR (recommended) |
| Mild MR (should be considered) |
| **Symptoms because of the MR** |
| Moderate or severe MR and EF >30% with no revascularisation possible (may be considered) |
| Moderate or severe MR and EF <30% and viability and revascularisation possible (should be considered) |

# 3 Echocardiography after mitral valve repair

See Table 8.10.

Table 8.10 Echocardiography after mitral valve repair

| Appearance of the mitral valve and annuloplasty ring |
| --- |
| Residual regurgitation:<br>• Grade<br>• Localisation (middle, medial, lateral)<br>• Through the valve or around the annuloplasty ring? |
| Presence and degree of stenosis |
| Systolic anterior motion of the anterior leaflet |
| LV outflow acceleration |
| LV size and function |
| RV size and function |
| Left atrial size |

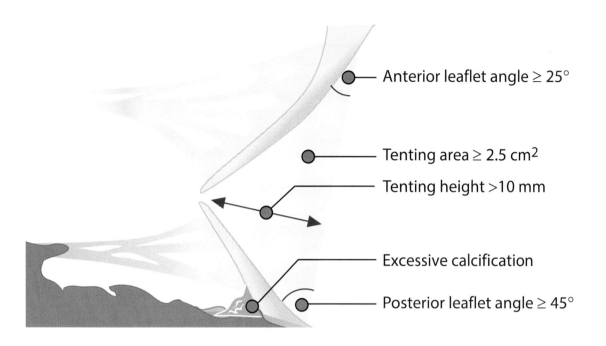

Anterior leaflet angle ≥ 25°

Tenting area ≥ 2.5 cm²

Tenting height >10 mm

Excessive calcification

Posterior leaflet angle ≥ 45°

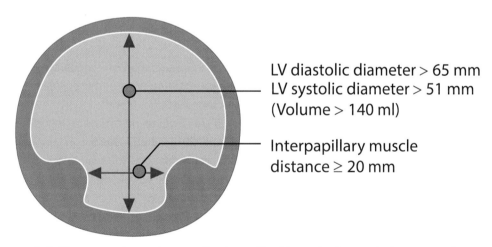

LV diastolic diameter > 65 mm
LV systolic diameter > 51 mm
(Volume > 140 ml)

Interpapillary muscle
distance ≥ 20 mm

Figure 8.8 Proposed markers of a low likelihood of repair in secondary (functional) mitral regurgitation.[13-17]

# References

1. Baumgartner H, Hung J, Bermejo J et al. Echocardiographic assessment of valve stenosis: EAE/ASE recommendations for clinical practice. *Eur J Echocardiogr* 2009;10:1–25.

2. Vahanian A, Alfieri O, Andreotti F et al. Guidelines on the management of valvular heart disease (version 2012). *Eur Heart J* 2012;33:2451–96.

3. Colombo T, Russo C, Ciliberto GR et al. Tricuspid regurgitation secondary to mitral valve disease: tricuspid annulus function as guide to tricuspid valve repair. *Cardiovasc Surg* 2001;9:369–77.

4. Dreyfus GD, Corbi PJ, Chan KM, Bahrami T. Secondary tricuspid regurgitation or dilatation: which should be the criteria for surgical repair? *Ann Thorac Surg* 2005;79:127–32.

5. Keenan NG, Cueff C, Cimidavella C et al. Usefulness of left atrial volume versus diameter to assess thromboembolic risk in mitral stenosis. *Am J Cardiol* 2010;106:1152–6.

6. Fawzy ME, Hegazy H, Shoukri M et al. Long-term clinical and echocardiographic results after successful balloon mitral valvotomy and predictors of long-term outcome. *Eur Heart J* 2005;26:1647–52.

7. Wilkins GT, Weyman AE, Abascal VM, Block PC, Palacios IF. Percutaneous balloon dilatation of the mitral valve: an analysis of echocardiographic variables related to outcome and the mechanism of dilatation. *Br Heart J* 1988;60:299–308.

8. Caldera I, van Herwerden LA, Taams MA, Bos E, Roelendt J. Multiplane transesophageal echocardiography and morphology of regurgitant mitral valves in surgical repair. *Eur Heart J* 1995;16:999–1006.

9. Lancellotti P, Tribouilloy C, Hagendorff A et al. European Association of Echocardiography recommendations for the assessment of valvular regurgitation. Part 2: mitral and tricuspid regurgitation (native valve disease). *Eur J Echocardiogr* 2010;11:307–32.

10. Nishimura RA, Otto CM, Bonow RO et al. 2014 AHA/ACC guideline for the management of patients with valvular heart disease. *J Am Coll Cardiol* 2014;63:e57–e185.

11. Zoghbi WA, Enriquez-Sarano M, Foster E et al. Recommendations for evaluation of the severity of native valvular regurgitation with two-dimensional and Doppler echocardiography. *J Am Soc Echocardiogr* 2003;16(7):777–802.

12. Lancellotti P, Troisfontaines P, Toussaunt AC, Pierard LA. Prognostic importance of exercise-induced changes in mitral regurgitation in patients with chronic ischaemic left ventricular dysfunction. *Circulation* 2003;108:1713–17.

13. Magne J, Pibarot P, Dagenais F, Hachicha Z, Dumesnil JG, Sénéchal M. Preoperative posterior leaflet angle accurately predicts outcome after restrictive mitral valve annuloplasty for ischaemic mitral regurgitation. *Circulation* 2007;115:782–91.

14. Calafiore AM, Gallina S, Di Mauro M et al. Mitral valve procedure in dilated cardiomyopathy: repair or replacement? *Ann Thorac Surg* 2001;71:1146–52.

15. Roshanali F, Mandegar MH, Yousefnia MA, Rayatzadeh H, Alaeddini F. A prospective study of predicting factors in ischaemic mitral regurgitation recurrence after ring annuloplasty. *Ann Thorac Surg* 2007;84:745–9.

16. Braun J, Bax JJ, Versteegh MI et al. Preoperative left ventricular dimensions predict reverse remodelling following restrictive mitral annuloplasty in ischaemic mitral regurgitation. *Eur J Cardiothorac Surg* 2005;27:847–53.
17. Grossi EA, Goldberg JD, LaPietra A et al. Ischaemic mitral reconstruction and replacement: comparison of long-term survival and complications. *J Thorac Cardiovasc Surg* 2001;122:1107–24.

# Right-sided valve disease

## 9

The right-sided valves should be assessed as part of the minimum standard protocol. Abnormalities are more likely if there is:

- left-sided disease
- RV dilatation, especially if the RV is also hyperdynamic.

## Tricuspid regurgitation

### 1 Is the valve morphologically normal?

- Trace or mild tricuspid regurgitation (TR) is seen in 80% of normal studies.
- Pathological tricuspid regurgitation is occasionally primary (caused by disease of the valve), but usually secondary (caused by disease of the myocardium or pulmonary hypertension) (Table 9.1).
- Examine the valve in all views (Figure 9.1).
  - Imaging all three leaflets may be aided by 3D.[1]
  - The normal apical displacement of the septal leaflet is up to 15 mm.
  - The whole annulus may be better imaged by 3D but normal ranges exist for 2D measured in systole:
    - 25–40 mm in the parasternal long-axis[2], and
    - 20–34 mm in the 4-chamber view.[3]
- RV dilatation from muscle disease, pulmonary hypertension or secondary to tricuspid regurgitation causes:
  - initially, annular dilatation with failure of leaflet coaptation
  - restriction of the leaflet tips as a result of further RV dilatation.

Table 9.1 Causes of tricuspid valve disease

| Cause | Notes |
|---|---|
| **Primary (10%)** | |
| Rheumatic disease | Doming without significant thickening<br>Commissural fusion may be more obvious on 3D<br>Associated left-sided rheumatic disease |
| Floppy valve | Eccentric jet directed away from the prolapsing leaflet<br>Often associated with mitral prolapse |

*(continued)*

Table 9.1 Causes of tricuspid valve disease (*continued*)

| Cause | Notes |
|---|---|
| Annular dilatation | May occur without prolapse<br>The normal annulus diameter is <40 mm (<21 mm/m$^2$)<br>(see Appendix 3, Table 3.1, page 220) |
| Endocarditis | In IV drug users or patients with indwelling cannulae |
| Carcinoid | Associated with pulmonary valve involvement<br>Fibrotic, stubby rigid leaflets |
| Congenital | Ebstein's anomaly (see Table 14.8, page 157) |
| Drugs | General thickening |
| Pacemaker | Regurgitation caused by: perforation; interference with closure; leaflet thickening or adhering to electrode |
| Trauma | Prolapse with ruptured chord |
| **Secondary (90%)** | |
| RV myopathy / RV infarct | Initially causes annular dilatation with failure of leaflet coaption. If severe, causes restriction of the leaflets. Look for associated left-sided myocardial abnormalities |
| Pulmonary hypertension | May be no abnormality of the leaflets unless there is secondary RV dilatation |

## 2 Grading tricuspid regurgitation

● Use all modalities available (Table 9.2). The most useful are the colour width and density of the continuous wave signal. Systolic flow reversal in the hepatic vein and IVC is a specific sign of severe TR.

● Trivial or mild tricuspid regurgitation is normal and could be noted in the text but should not appear in the conclusion of the report.

Table 9.2 Grading tricuspid regurgitation[4, 5]

| | Mild | Moderate | Severe |
|---|---|---|---|
| Colour neck (mm) | Usually none | <7 | ≥7 |
| PISA radius (mm) | <5 | 6–9 | >9 |
| EROA (mm$^2$) | – | – | ≥40* |
| Regurgitant vol (ml) | – | – | ≥45* |
| Continuous wave | Incomplete | Low or moderate intensity | Dense and may be triangular (Figure 9.1) |
| Hepatic vein flow | Normal | Maybe systolic blunting | Systolic reversal (Figure 9.2) |

*Not routinely performed

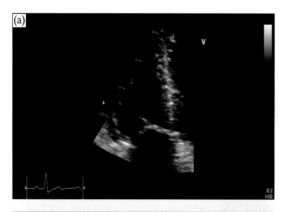

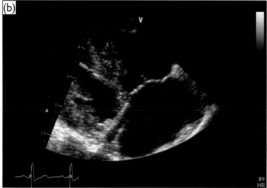

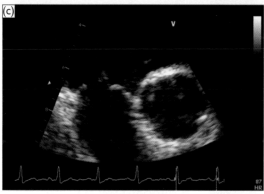

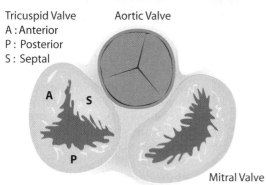

Tricuspid Valve
A : Anterior
P : Posterior
S : Septal

Aortic Valve

Mitral Valve

**Figure 9.1 The normal tricuspid valve.** The diagram shows the leaflets and helps understand the leaflets imaged in the main views. The 4-chamber view (a) shows the anterior (left) and septal (right) leaflets. The parasternal long-axis view (b) shows the anterior (right) and either septal or posterior leaflet (left) depending on whether the septum or posterior LV wall is imaged. The short-axis view (c) shows the septal or anterior leaflet (right) and the anterior or posterior leaflet (left) depending on the cut.

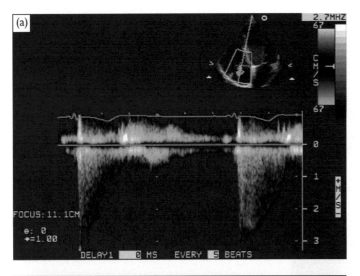

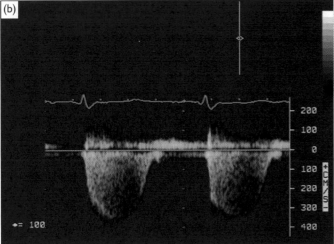

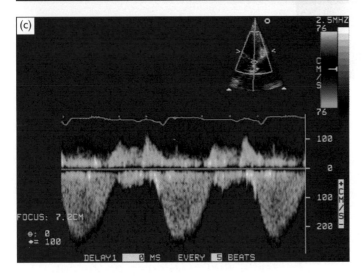

**Figure 9.2 Continuous wave signal in tricuspid regurgitation.** Mild regurgitation causes a dagger-shaped, low-intensity signal (a). Moderate regurgitation causes a large intra-atrial jet on colour mapping with a complete continuous wave signal (b). Severe regurgitation has a dense signal which initially retains its usual shape but, when very severe, the continuous wave signal (c) may be dagger-shaped.

## 3 Describe RV size and function

See also Chapter 5.

- Progressive RV dilatation and reduction in systolic function are indications for surgery even without symptoms.[6]
- Early repair is recommended with a flail tricuspid leaflet after trauma if the RV is significantly dilated at the initial assessment but no thresholds are available.[7]

## 4 Estimate pulmonary artery pressure

See Chapter 6.

## 5 Echocardiography and surgery

- Indications for surgery are severe TR with symptoms, or as in Table 9.3.
- The type of surgery is guided by echocardiography:
  - Annular dilatation usually responds to annuloplasty.
  - Severe systolic restriction usually requires more advanced repair techniques or valve replacement.
  - Tricuspid prolapse may be repairable.
- Severe thickening usually requires replacement.

Table 9.3 Echocardiographic indications for surgery in tricuspid regurgitation

| Having left-sided surgery |
| --- |
| Moderate or severe TR |
| Tricuspid annulus $\geqslant 40$ mm ($\geqslant 21$ mm/m$^2$) and either mild TR (rheumatic disease) or moderate/severe (associated with mitral prolapse) |
| **Isolated severe TR and no symptoms** |
| Progressive RV dilatation |
| Progressive reduction in RV function |

# Tricuspid stenosis

## 1 Valve appearance

- Tricuspid stenosis is usually rheumatic but may also be congenital (Ebstein, tricuspid atresia), or occur in carcinoid or as a result of dense fibrosis secondary to SLE or multiple pacemaker electrodes.

## 2 Recognising tricuspid stenosis

- Restriction of the leaflets (Figure 9.3) may not be obvious on imaging. Tricuspid stenosis is suggested if:
  - $V_{max}$ >1.0 m/s (or more likely >1.5 m/s)[8] or
  - mean gradient >2 mmHg[9, 10]
- Another clue is a small right ventricle (because of underfilling) and large right atrium (because of high back pressure).
- Signs suggesting severe stenosis are:
  - mean gradient ≥5 mmHg
  - pressure half-time ≥190 ms.

## 3 Surgery

- Surgery is indicated for severe tricuspid stenosis and symptoms or is performed at the time of surgery for coexistent left-sided disease.

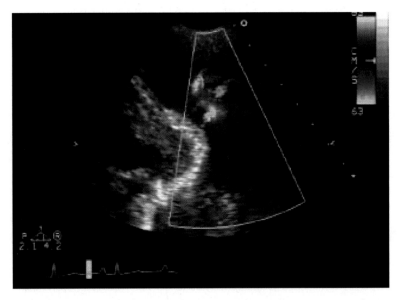

**Figure 9.3 Tricuspid stenosis.** Tricuspid stenosis may be missed because, unlike the situation with the mitral valve, there is little thickening or calcification.

 MISTAKES TO AVOID

- A rheumatic TV is easily missed because the leaflets can be thin. Lone rheumatic TV disease is extremely unusual so a useful prompt to check the TV carefully is a rheumatic MV

## CHECKLIST FOR REPORTING TRICUSPID VALVE DISEASE

1. Tricuspid valve appearance and movement:
   a. Bowing
   b. Failure of leaflet tips to appose
   c. Prolapse
2. Grade of regurgitation
3. Transtricuspid gradient if valve restricted
4. RV size and function
5. PA pressure
6. Left-sided valves

# Pulmonary stenosis and regurgitation

- Pulmonary stenosis (PS) is almost always congenital (Table 9.4). It may be part of more complex cardiac lesions, especially tetralogy of Fallot, or associated with other lesions, e.g. ASD. It may also be associated with more general congenital syndromes (Noonan, Williams, LEOPARD – see Table 14.1, page 149)
- The obstruction is at valve level in 90%, and is subvalvar in 5%, supravalvar in 1% and in a branch in 5%

Table 9.4 Causes of pulmonary valve disease

| **Pulmonary stenosis** |
| --- |
| Congenital |
| Carcinoid |
| **Pulmonary regurgitation** |
| Prior intervention for congenital stenosis |
| Endocarditis |
| Functional:<br>• Pulmonary hypertension<br>• PA or annular dilatation |
| Carcinoid |

# 1 Appearance of the valve

- Use all views available: parasternal long-axis and short-axis, modified 5-chamber, subcostal.
- An initial clue to the presence of stenosis is turbulent flow in the RV outflow tract during systole on colour Doppler mapping.
- A stenotic valve is:
  - either dysplastic and thickened (e.g. in Noonan Syndrome); or
  - relatively thin, but with systolic bowing and therefore visible in systole as well as diastole.

# 2 Is there pulmonary regurgitation?

- Trace or mild regurgitation is normal. A jet originating near the edge of the orifice should not be mistaken for coronary artery flow.
- Severe pulmonary regurgitation (PR) is suggested by the findings in Table 9.5.

**Table 9.5** Factors suggesting severe pulmonary regurgitation

| |
| --- |
| A wide colour jet (e.g. >7.5 mm or >50% of the RV outflow tract)[11] |
| Diastolic flow reversal visible in the distal main pulmonary artery or branches (Figure 9.4) |
| A steep dense signal (pressure half-time <100 ms)[12, 13] (Figure 9.5) |
| Ratio of PR duration:diastolic duration[14] <0.77 |
| Dilated, active RV |

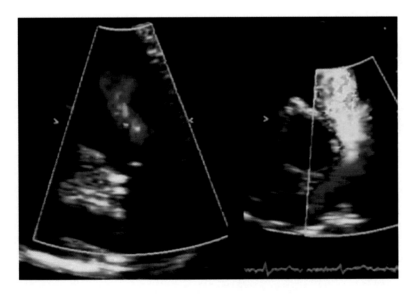

Figure 9.4 Pulmonary regurgitation – colour map. Mild regurgitation is shown on the left with a narrow jet originating at the valve level. Severe regurgitation on the right has a jet filling the RV outflow tract with flow reversal as far as the right pulmonary artery branch.

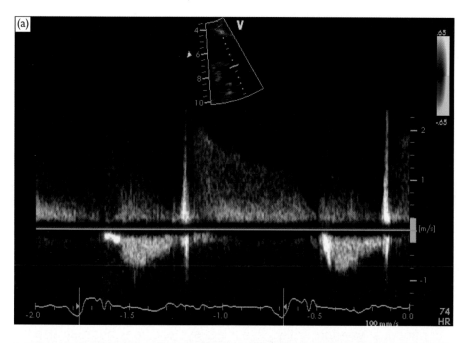

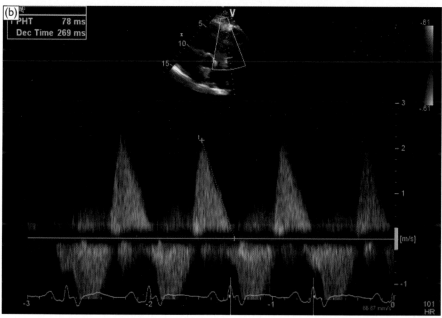

Figure 9.5 Pulmonary regurgitation – continuous wave signal. In normal mild PR the signal has a slow descent (a) while in severe regurgitation (b) the pressure half-time is <100 ms, 78 ms in this example.

And here's an electronic link to a loop on the website or use
http://goo.gl/eQmasZ

## 3 What is the pressure difference across the valve?

The main method of grading is by the transpulmonary $V_{max}$ (Table 9.6). Severe stenosis is suggested by:[15, 16]

- transpulmonary $V_{max}$ >4.0 m/s
- mean pressure difference >50 mmHg
- mean pressure difference <50 mmHg with RV dysfunction.

Table 9.6 Grading pulmonary stenosis

|  | Mild | Moderate | Severe |
|---|---|---|---|
| $V_{max}$ (m/s) | <3.0 | 3.0–4.0 | >4.0 |

## 4 Check the level of the obstruction

- A muscular obstruction in the RV outflow tract (infundibulum) or midcavity (double-chamber RV) may be mistaken for or be associated with pulmonary valve stenosis.
  - The continuous waveform may have a late systolic peak but may also be identical to obstruction at valve level.
  - Pulsed Doppler may identify the level of obstruction.
  - The diagnosis may require CMR if the echocardiographic image quality is suboptimal.
- A pulmonary artery membrane may also be mistaken for valvar obstruction but is rare.

## 5 What is the pulmonary artery pressure?

See also Chapter 6.
- Dominant pulmonary regurgitation may be caused by pulmonary hypertension.
- Pulmonary stenosis protects the pulmonary circulation against the effect of high flow from a left-to-right shunt.

## 6 Assess the pulmonary artery

Look for dilatation of the main and branch pulmonary arteries (Table 9.7).

Table 9.7 Normal pulmonary artery dimensions[17]

| Pulmonary artery | Measurement (mm) |
|---|---|
| RV outflow diameter | 18–34 |
| PV annulus | 10–22 |

| Pulmonary artery | Measurement (mm) |
|---|---|
| Main pulmonary artery | 9–29 |
| Right pulmonary branch | 7–17 |
| Left pulmonary branch | 6–14 |

## 7 Assess right ventricular size and function

See Chapter 5.

## 8 Other techniques

Once severe pulmonary valve disease is detected by echocardiography, CMR is used to:

- quantify the degree of pulmonary regurgitation – a regurgitant volume of >40 ml/beat and a regurgitant fraction >35% are taken as severe
- measure RV volumes for serial studies
- assess the RV outflow tract and differentiate double-chamber RV from infundibular stenosis
- assess branch pulmonary artery stenosis including lung perfusion.

## 9 Are there indications for invasive intervention?

- Intervention is indicated for severe PS or PR and symptoms or reduced exercise tolerance.
- Echocardiographic indications for surgery in asymptomatic patients are given in Tables 9.8 and 9.9.
- The intervention of choice for valvar PS is balloon valvotomy; for PR it is valve replacement.

Table 9.8 Echocardiographic indications for surgery in asymptomatic PS[18]

| |
|---|
| RV outflow obstruction with $V_{max}$ >4.0 m/s if repairable |
| If unrepairable, TR $V_{max}$ >4.3 m/s |
| $V_{max}$ <4.0 m/s and<br>• decreased RV systolic function<br>• double-chambered RV<br>or<br>• right-to-left shunting via an ASD or VSD |
| Peripheral PS with >50% diameter narrowing and RV systolic pressure >50 mmHg |

Table 9.9 Indications for surgery in asymptomatic severe PR[6, 18]

| |
|---|
| RV EF <40% on CMR |
| Progressive RV dilatation on CMR ($\geqslant$160 ml/m² in diastole or $\geqslant$82 ml/m² in systole) |
| Moderate or worse functional TR as a result of progressive RV dilatation |
| Another lesion requiring surgery |

 MISTAKES TO AVOID

- Do not use the TR $V_{max}$ alone to calculate PA systolic pressure if there is pulmonary stenosis or other RV outflow obstruction. Subtracting the $4V_{pulm}^2$ from $4V_{tr}$ will give a better estimate
- Missing severe pulmonary regurgitation because the diastolic jet may be wide and low momentum

### CHECKLIST FOR REPORTING PULMONARY VALVE DISEASE

1. Appearance and motion of the pulmonary valve
2. $V_{max}$, and mean gradient
3. Grade of pulmonary regurgitation
4. RV size, morphology and systolic function
5. Diameter of pulmonary artery
6. Estimated PA systolic pressure

## References

1. Badano LP, Agricola E, de Isla LP, Gianfagna P, Zamorano JL. Evaluation of the tricuspid valve morphology and function by transthoracic real-time three-dimensional echocardiography. *Eur J Echocardiogr* 2009;10:477–84.
2. Foale R, Nihoyannopoulos P, McKenna W et al. Echocardiographic measurements of the normal adult right ventricle. *Br Heart J* 1986; 56: 33–44.
3. Dwivedi G, Mahadevan G, Jimenez D, Frenneaux M, Steeds R. Reference values for mitral and tricuspid annular dimensions using two-dimensional echocardiography. *Echo Research and Practice* published September 1, 2014, doi:10.1530/ERP-14-0062.
4. Zoghbi WA, Enriquez-Sarano M, Foster E et al. Recommendations for evaluation of the severity of native valvular regurgitation with two-dimensional and Doppler echocardiography. *J Am Soc Echocardiogr* 2003;16(7):777–802.

5.  Lancellotti P, Tribouilloy C, Hagendorff A et al. European Association of Echocardiography recommendations for the assessment of valvular regurgitation. Part 2: mitral and tricuspid regurgitation (native valve disease). *Eur J Echocardiogr* 2010;11:307–32.
6.  Vahanian A, Alfieri O, Andreotti F et al. Guidelines on the management of valvular heart disease (version 2012). *Eur Heart J* 2012;33:2451–96.
7.  Messika-Zeitoun D, Thomson H, Bellamy M, Scott C, Tribouilloy C, Dearani J, Tajik AJ, Schaff H, Enriquez-Sarano M. Medical and surgical outcome of tricuspid regurgitation caused by flail leaflets. *J Thorac Cardiovasc Surg* 2004;128:296–302.
8.  Parris TM, Panidis JP, Ross J, Mintz GS. Doppler echocardiographic findings in rheumatic tricuspid stenosis. *Am J Cardiol* 1987;60(16):1414–16.
9.  Ribeiro PA, Al Zaibag M, Al Kasab S et al. Provocation and amplification of the transvalvular pressure gradient in rheumatic tricuspid stenosis. *Am J Cardiol* 1988;61(15):1307–11.
10. Fawzy ME, Mercer EN, Dunn B, Al-Amri M, Andaya W. Doppler echocardiography in the evaluation of tricuspid stenosis. *Eur Heart J* 1989;10:985–90.
11. Puchalski MD, Askovich B, Sower CT, Williams RV, Minicch LL, Tani LY. Pulmonary regurgitation: determining severity by echocardiography and magnetic resonance imaging. *Cong Heart Dis* 2008;3:168–75.
12. Silversides CK, Veldtman GR, Crossin J et al. Pressure half time predicts hemodynamically significant pulmonary regurgitation in adult patients with repaired tetralogy of Fallot. *J Am Soc Echocardiogr* 2003;16:1057–62.
13. Yang H, Pu M, Chambers CE, Weber HS, Myers JL, Davidson WR. Quantitative assessment of pulmonary insufficiency by Doppler echocardiography in patients with adult congenital heart disease. *J Am Soc Echocardiogr* 2008;16:157–64.
14. Van der Zwaan HB, Geleijnse ML, McGhie JS et al. Right ventricular quantification in clinical practice: two-dimension vs three-dimensional echocardiography compared with cardiac magnetic resonance imaging. *Eur J Echocardiogr* 2011;12:656–64.
15. Silvilairat S, Cabalka AK, Cetta F, Hagler DJ, O'Leary PW. Echocardiographic assessment of isolated pulmonary valve stenosis: which outpatient Doppler gradient has the most clinical validity? *J Am Soc Echocardiogr* 2005;18(11):1137–42.
16. Baumgartner H, Bonhoeffer P, De Groot NMS et al. ESC guidelines for the management of grown-up congenital heart disease: The Task Force on the Management of Grown-up Congenital Heart Disease of the European Society of Cardiology (ESC). *Eur Heart J* 2010;31:2915–57.
17. Triulzi MO, Gillam LD, Gentile F. Normal adult cross-sectional echocardiographic values: linear dimensions and chamber areas. *Echocardiography* 1984;1:403–26.
18. Nishimura RA, Otto CM, Bonow RO, et al. 2014 AHA/ACC guideline for the management of patients with valvular heart disease. *J Am Coll Cardiol* 2014;63:e57–e185.

# Replacement heart valves

10

## General

- Replacement valves are usually obstructive compared to a normal native valve and it is important to differentiate normal from pathological obstruction.
- Minor regurgitation through the valve is usually normal and the pattern differs between the types of valve.

### 1 Types of valve

- Conventional replacement valves are either biological or mechanical.
- The most frequently implanted biological types are those made from animal tissue, 'xenografts' (Table 10.1a and b).[1] These are usually made from pig aortic valves or bovine pericardium and consist of a stent surrounded by a sewing ring with the valve cusps inside.
- Stentless xenograft valves were introduced in the hope of improving haemodynamic function, durability and complications (Figure 10.1c). They are less frequently implanted now but still require echocardiography.
- Homografts ('allografts') are human valves and are implanted in the young with the hope of longer durability than xenografts and because anticoagulation is not needed. They are also used in patients with endocarditis.
- The Ross procedure involves autotransplanting the patient's pulmonary valve to the aortic position and replacing it with a homograft. This means that a living valve is in the aortic position while a preserved valve is in the lower-pressure right side. Echocardiography is required of both autograft and pulmonary homograft.
- Sutureless valves were developed to speed up the implantation process to limit bypass time in high-risk patients and to facilitate minimally invasive access. These are not yet used routinely.
- An important new class of valve is the transcatheter valve. There are many available or in production but the most commonly implanted are the Edwards SAPIEN (Figure 10.1g) and the Medtronic Corevalve (Figure 10.1h).
- The most frequently implanted mechanical valve now (Table 10.1b) is the bileaflet mechanical valve (Figure 10.1d and e), but tilting disc valves are still used (Figure 10.1f) and caged-ball valves will still require echocardiography. Bileaflet valves are not 'metal' but usually made from pyrolytic carbon.

Table 10.1a Biological xenograft valves

| Type | Makes |
|---|---|
| **Stented xenograft** | |
| Porcine | C-E SAV, C-E Duraflex, Mosaic, Epic, Hancock, SJM Biocor, Labcor porcine |
| Pericardial | Perimount, Mitroflow, Labcor pericardial, Biocor pericardial, Trifecta, C-E Biophysio, Sorin More, Sorin Soprano |
| Sutureless | Perceval S, Edwards Intuity, 3F Enable, Trilogy |
| Transcatheter | SAPIEN, Corevalve, Jena, Portico |
| **Stentless** | |
| Porcine | Toronto*, Medtronic Freestyle, Cryolife-O'Brien,* Koehler Elan, Labcor stentless, Edwards Prima, Biocor |
| Pericardial | Freedom Solo, Pericarbon |

C-E: Carpentier-Edwards; SJM: St Jude Medical
*Now withdrawn

Table 10.1b Mechanical replacement valves

| Type | Makes |
|---|---|
| Caged-ball | Starr-Edwards |
| Tilting disc | Björk-Shiley, Medtronic Hall, Sorin Allcarbon, Omnicarbon, Koehler Ultracor |
| Bileaflet | St Jude, Carbomedics, On-X, Sorin bicarbon, ATS, Medtronic Advantage, Edwards Mira |

# 2 Complications of replacement heart valves

Patients may present with symptoms as a result of:

- dysfunction of the replacement valve
- endocarditis
- other disease: LV or RV dysfunction or other valve disease.

Echocardiography is important in differentiating these causes. The complications of replacement valves (Table 10.2) may cause regurgitation or obstruction.

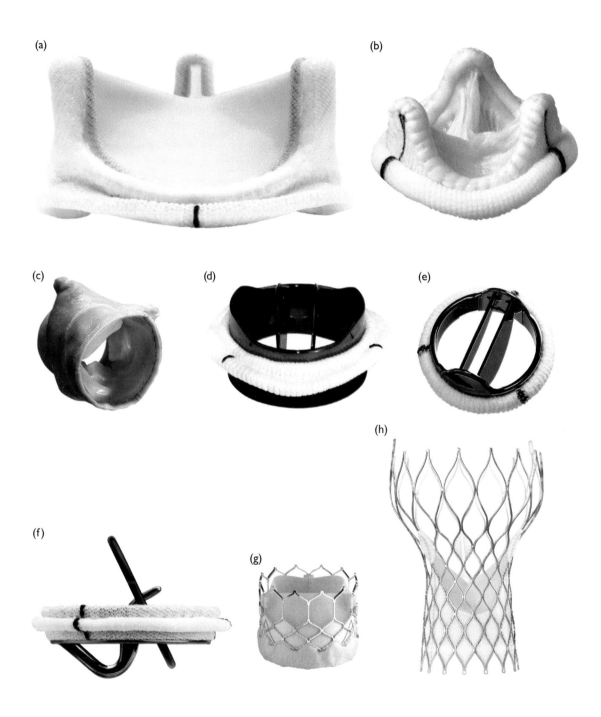

Figure 10.1 Images of replacement heart valves:
**Stented biological valves:** (a) Magna-Ease (bovine pericardial), (b) Epic (porcine).
**Stentless biological valve:** (c) Medtronic Freestyle.
**Bileaflet mechanical mitral valve:** (d) OnX, (e) Master HP.
**Single tilting disc:** (f) Medtronic-Hall.
**Transcatheter:** (g) Edwards SAPIEN, (h) Medtronic Corevalve (Reproduced by permission of Edwards Lifesciences Corp, Medtronic, OnX and St Jude Medical).

Table 10.2 Complications of replacement heart valves

| Complication | Mechanical | Biological | Echocardiographic effect |
|---|---|---|---|
| Primary failure | – | +++ | Thickened cusps with regurgitation >> stenosis |
| Thrombosis | +++ | + | Obstruction |
| Thromboembolism | +++ | ++ | Nil |
| Infection | ++ | ++ | Vegetations, abscess, dehiscence |
| Pannus | + | + | Obstruction of closure or opening of leaflet. May be intermittent |
| Dehiscence | ++ | ++ | Paraprosthetic regurgitation |
| Bleeding | +++ | + | Nil |

## 3 LV and RV function and pulmonary artery pressure

- A hyperdynamic LV is a clue that there is severe prosthetic aortic or mitral regurgitation.
- A rise in pulmonary artery pressure can be a sign of prosthetic mitral valve dysfunction.

## 4 When is TOE indicated?

TTE and TOE are complementary and TOE is rarely used without initial TTE (Table 10.3). Although TOE is usually necessary to image vegetations and posterior root abscesses, anterior root abscesses may be better seen transthoracically.

Table 10.3 Indications for TOE

| |
|---|
| Endocarditis clinically likely |
| Obstruction suggested by TTE to:<br>• image leaflets, or<br>• detect thrombus, pannus or vegetations |
| To image leaflet opening to differentiate patient prosthesis mismatch from pathological obstruction in an aortic valve replacement |
| Haemolysis (small regurgitant jet often not detected on TTE) |
| Symptomatic patient and suboptimal TTE imaging |
| Paraprosthetic mitral regurgitation of uncertain severity |
| Thromboembolism despite therapeutic INR (to detect pannus or thrombus) |

# Replacement valves in the aortic position

## 1 Do the leaflets and valve appear normal?

- The cusps of a biological valve should be thin (<3 mm) and should open fully.
- In a parasternal long-axis view, the tips of the leaflets of a bileaflet mechanical valve will be seen in systole beyond the housing if the valve is placed horizontally. On M-mode they often flutter slightly.
- A tilting disc or ball may appear as an indistinct mass in a parasternal long-axis view and may be difficult to tell apart; the cage of a caged-ball valve is usually better seen in an apical long-axis view.
- As an adjunct to imaging, colour filling the outflow tract and the orifice of the valve in all views suggests normal function.
- The valve should not rock, which implies a large paraprosthetic leak.
- Stentless valves may be associated with a thickened aortic root caused by oedema and haematoma which gradually resolves over the first 6 months after implantation. For other valves, major or asymmetric thickening or echolucent pockets raise the possibility of endocarditis.

## 2 Colour Doppler – regurgitation

- All mechanical valves have 'physiological' regurgitation through the valve which may occur only during closing or after closure or throughout diastole (Figure 10.2). Trivial or mild regurgitation across the valve occurs in about 10% of normal biological valves.
- To establish whether the regurgitation is normal or pathological it is necessary to determine its origin and grade and whether there is thickening of the cusps.

### 2.1 Origin of the jet

- How many jets are there, and are they through the valve (Figure 10.2), paraprosthetic (Figure 10.3) or both? Localisation can only be certain if the base or neck of the jet can be imaged in relation to the sewing ring.
- For a mechanical valve, the jets through the valve should match the typical pattern expected of the design (Figure 10.2).
- Regurgitation through the valve in bileaflet mechanical valves ('pivotal washing jets') begins close to the edge of the orifice and must not be mistaken for paraprosthetic jets.
- The site of a paraprosthetic aortic jet can be described on the sewing ring as a clock face in the parasternal short-axis view.
- Mild regurgitation through a biological valve associated with a thickened cusp is an early sign of primary failure, especially if either the regurgitation or thickening increases on serial studies.

**Long Axis**    **Short Axis**

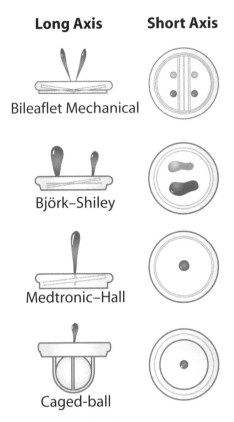

Bileaflet Mechanical

Björk–Shiley

Medtronic–Hall

Caged-ball

**Figure 10.2** Patterns of normal regurgitation.

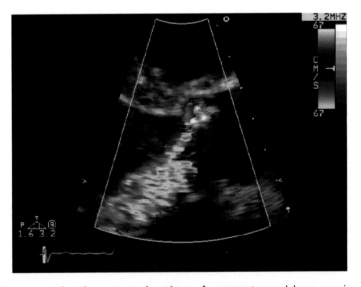

**Figure 10.3 Paraprosthetic regurgitation.** A parasternal long-axis view of a bileaflet mechanical aortic valve. There is a jet originating in the aorta with the neck clearly imaged outside the sewing ring and directed eccentrically in the LV outflow tract.

## 2.2 Severity of regurgitation

- Normal regurgitation through a mechanical valve is usually low in momentum (relatively homogeneous colour) with an incomplete or very low-intensity continuous wave (CW) signal.
- For larger jets, use the same methods as for native regurgitation (see page 68–71). Assessing the height of a jet relative to LV outflow diameter may be difficult since paraprosthetic jets are often eccentric.
- The circumference of the sewing ring occupied by the aortic jet is another guide: mild (<10%), moderate (10–20%), severe (>20%). This is less reliable if there are multiple jets as may occur with a TAVI.

# 3 Spectral Doppler

- Steerable CW from the apex is sufficient if the patient is well and the valve clearly normal but, if there is doubt, the stand-alone probe should be used in at least two windows as for native aortic stenosis.
- It is important not to position the pulsed sample too close to the replacement valve as this results in an artefactually high EOA.
- The minimum dataset is $V_{max}$, mean gradient and EOA using the continuity equation.[2]
- High velocities are frequently found and are caused by:
  - pathological obstruction (see section 4 below)
  - patient prosthesis mismatch (see section 5 below).

# 4 Is there evidence of obstruction?

- There are definitive signs of obstruction (Table 10.4):
  - Thickened and immobile biological cusps
  - Stuck leaflet. The disk or leaflets of an obstructed mechanical valve may be difficult to image parasternally, but may be seen more easily from the apical 5-chamber and long-axis views
  - A narrowed colour flow map complements the imaging
  - If imaging is still difficult, the possibilities are:
    - TOE but leaflets of a mechanical valve may still be difficult to image
    - Fluoroscopy, which is widely available in the catheter lab
    - CT which may also be able to image pannus.
- Compare the $V_{max}$ velocity, mean gradient and EOA by the continuity equation with normal values for type and size (Appendix 3, Tables A3.5–3.6, pages 223–225) and/or with previous studies in the same patient. Obstruction is corroborated or suggested by a difference from these. A difference of 25% from previous studies is used as an arbitrary cut-point allowing for measurement error.

Table 10.4 When to suspect aortic valve obstruction

| Thickened or immobile cusps or occluder |
| --- |
| Narrowed colour map |
| Measurements outside normal values (Appendix 3, Tables A3.5–A3.6) |
| Change in measurements by more than about 25% on serial studies |
| In the absence of serial studies, suspect if:[2]<br>• $V_{max}$ >4.0 ms<br>• mean pressure difference >35 mmHg<br>• EOA <0.8 cm$^2$<br>• acceleration time >100 ms* |

*Time from start of systolic signal to $V_{max}$

## 5 Patient-prosthesis mismatch

● This means that the valve is functioning normally but is too small for the size of the patient.
● Although it has been associated with an increased risk of events and of slower regression of LV hypertrophy, it is only a practical clinical problem if the patient is symptomatic usually with breathlessness.
● It is defined by:
  ● an indexed EOA <0.85 cm$^2$/m$^2$ (severe if <0.6 cm$^2$/m$^2$)
  ● indexed EOA, $V_{max}$ and mean gradient in the normal range for the types and size of valve
  ● normal cusp and leaflet opening.

## 6 Signs of early failure

● Third generation stented biological valves in the aortic position tend to fail from about 7 years[3] and guidelines suggest routine annual echocardiography from 10 years after implantation.[4]
● The failure mode varies according to the valve design, but stented valves often develop small tears near the cusp base. On echo this shows as thickening associated with an initially small jet of regurgitation.

## 7 TAVI

● The assessment of TAVI valves is similar to other designs of replacement valve.[5]
● Lack of durability data means that regular assessment at least annually is necessary to detect possible early failure.
● There may be flow acceleration in the stent proximal to the cusps. If the pulsed sample is placed too far into the LV outflow tract, there may be an erroneously high estimate of EOA.

- Even mild paraprosthetic regurgitation may be associated with a high risk of events. These may be multiple and associated with regurgitation through the valve.

 **MISTAKES TO AVOID**

- Normal regurgitant jets in bileaflet mechanical valves begin close to the edge of the orifice and must not be mistaken for paraprosthetic jets
- Overdiagnosing obstruction with a single high $V_{max}$

**CHECKLIST FOR REPORTING REPLACEMENT AORTIC VALVES**

1. Appearance of the valve
2. $V_{max}$, mean gradient and EOA
3. Presence, location and grade of regurgitation
4. If velocities and gradients high:
   a. Is there evidence of pathological obstruction?
   b. Is there patient-prosthesis mismatch?
5. LV size and function:
   a. Dilated and hyperdynamic with severe aortic (or mitral) regurgitation
   b. Newly dilated and hypokinetic with severe aortic stenosis
6. Aorta:
   a. Size of ascending aorta
   b. Evidence of coarctation if the valve replacement was for a bicuspid aortic valve

# Replacement valves in the mitral position

## 1 Do the leaflets and valve appear normal?

- Biological cusps and mechanical leaflets are more easily imaged than for the aortic position.
- Some appearances which are normal but can cause confusion are:
  - the leaflets of a bileaflet mechanical valve may shut at slightly different rates
  - cavitations (bubbles) in the LV which occur with all types of valve but especially bileaflet mechanical valves

- if the surgeon has retained chordae, the valve may rock slightly
- fibrin strands attached to the valve (seen best on TOE).
- Colour mapping filling the orifice in all views during diastole is a useful corroboration of normal opening.

## 2 Is there regurgitation?

- An easily seen jet is usually paraprosthetic since normal transprosthetic regurgitation tends to be hidden by flow shielding (unless the left atrium is very large).
- The intraventricular flow recruitment region of paraprosthetic regurgitation can usually be seen even when the intra-atrial jet is invisible. This allows the regurgitation to be localised using the sewing ring as a clock face.

## 3 Severity of mitral prosthetic regurgitation

- Severe paraprosthetic regurgitation may be obvious from:
  - a large region of flow convergence within the LV
  - a broad neck
  - a hyperdynamic left ventricle
  - a dense continuous wave signal especially with early depressurisation (dagger shape).
- If there is doubt, transoesophageal echocardiography is necessary to evaluate jet width, the size of the intra-atrial jet and pulmonary vein flow (looking for systolic flow reversal).

## 4 Is there evidence of obstruction?

See Table 10.5.

- Most information for the diagnosis of obstruction is found from imaging and colour flow mapping.
- Measure peak velocity and mean gradient and compare to normal values (Appendix 3, Table A3.7).
- Pressure half-time does not reflect orifice area in normally functioning prosthetic mitral valves and the Hatle orifice area formula (Appendix 4, section A4.3) is not valid. However, the pressure half-time lengthens significantly when the valve becomes obstructed (Figure 10.4).
- The effective orifice area is not routinely calculated. However, if the patient remains breathless or the pulmonary artery pressure fails to normalise after surgery despite a normal or equivocal mean gradient, effective area can be calculated as:
  - stroke volume in the LV outflow tract / transmitral velocity integral.

- Patient-prosthesis mismatch is defined by an indexed effective orifice area:
  - moderate 0.9–1.2 cm²/m²
  - severe <0.9 cm²/m².

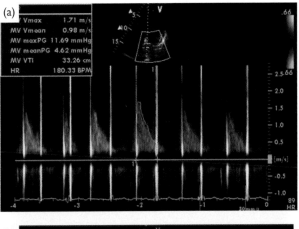

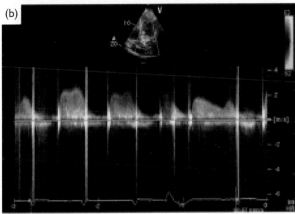

**Figure 10.4 Transmitral Doppler signal:** (a) soon after implantation with a pressure half-time 50 ms, and (b) after stopping warfarin on admission in pulmonary oedema with a pressure half-time 350 ms.

**Table 10.5** When to suspect mitral obstruction[2]

| |
| --- |
| Thickened and immobile cusps or occluder |
| Narrowed colour inflow |
| Pressure half-time >200 ms with $V_{max}$ ≥2.5 m/s |
| Change in measurements by more than about 25% from previous study |
| Increase in pulmonary artery pressure |
| EOA <1.0 cm² |
| $VTI_{mv}/VTI_{LVOT}$ >2.5 |

**MISTAKES TO AVOID**

- Shielding can make it difficult to see regurgitant jets in the LA so check for flow convergence at the origin of the jet within the LV and use off-axis views
- Not responding to a hyperdynamic LV as an indirect sign of severe paraprosthetic regurgitation
- Not doing a TOE to look for a small paraprosthetic jet if there is clinically severe haemolysis

## CHECKLIST FOR REPORTING MITRAL REPLACEMENT VALVES

1. Appearance of the valve
2. $V_{max}$, mean gradient and pressure half-time
3. Presence, location and grade of regurgitation
4. Evidence of obstruction
5. LV size and function:
   a. Dilated and hyperdynamic with severe mitral regurgitation
   b. Small in severe mitral stenosis
6. RV size and pulmonary pressures

# Replacement valves in the tricuspid position

## 1 Does the valve appear normal?

Use all views. The modified parasternal long-axis view often gives excellent views of the tricuspid valve. Normality is established by:

- normal thickness and movement of the biological cusps or mechanical leaflets
- colour map fills the orifice in all views
- no rocking of the valve (as a sign of dehiscence)
- no extraneous masses (suggesting vegetations or thrombus).

## 2 Is there regurgitation?

- Is this through the valve, paraprosthetic or both?
- Regurgitation is graded as for native tricuspid valve regurgitation. A jet width >7 mm suggests severe regurgitation.
- Look for flow reversal in the hepatic vein and a hyperdynamic RV as indirect signs of severe regurgitation.

## 3 Is there evidence of obstruction?

See Figure 10.5.

- Thrombosis of right-sided mechanical replacements is more common than for left-sided valves.
- The minimum data set is $V_{max}$, mean gradient and pressure half-time. Because of respiratory variability, measurements should be made over 3–5 cycles even in sinus rhythm (Table 10.6).
- Primary failure of a biological valve is usually obvious transthoracically. Confirming the cause of obstruction of a mechanical valve usually requires TOE.
- Thrombolysis is the first-line treatment for thrombosis whatever the size of the thrombus in contradistinction to left-sided thrombosis.

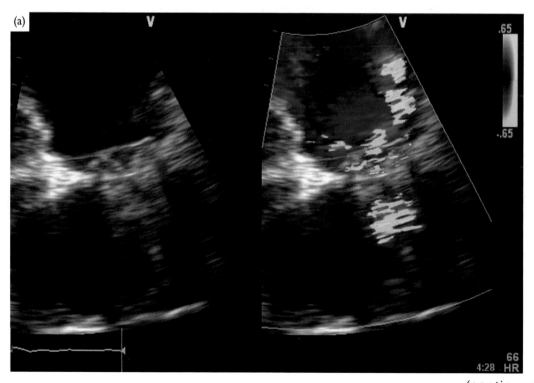

*(continued)*

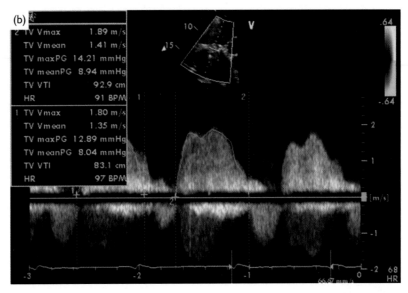

Figure 10.5 Obstructed bileaflet mechanical valve in the tricuspid position. (a) shows the leaflets stuck half open and in (b), the continuous wave signal shows a mean gradient of between 8 and 9 mmHg.

Table 10.6 When to suspect obstruction of a replacement tricuspid valve[2, 6, 7]

| |
|---|
| Thickened and immobile cusps or occluder |
| Narrowed colour inflow |
| Dilated IVC or right atrium |
| Peak velocity >1.6 m/s (in the absence of severe tricuspid regurgitation) |
| Mean gradient >6 mmHg |
| Pressure half-time >230 ms |

# Replacement valves in the pulmonary position

Pulmonary stenosis is often treated percutaneously. Replacement valves may be used:

- to correct severe regurgitation after percutaneous dilatation of a stenotic valve, e.g. in tetralogy of Fallot
- to replace the harvested native pulmonary valve during a Ross procedure.

## 1 Does the valve appear normal?

Imaging the valve leaflets may be difficult. Use all views including subcostal.

## 2 Is there regurgitation?

This is graded as for native regurgitation (Table 9.5, page 102).

## 3 Is there evidence of obstruction?

See Table 10.7.

- A serial change is more reliable than a single measurement. Published normal ranges are derived from small populations.
- New or progressive RV dysfunction is a further indirect sign of valve pathology. Long-axis excursion and tissue Doppler systolic velocity are always reduced after any cardiac surgery.

Table 10.7 When to suspect pulmonary obstruction[2, 8]

| |
|---|
| Cusp thickening or immobility |
| Narrowing of colour flow |
| Peak velocity above 2 m/s for homograft and 3 m/s for all other valve types (suspicious, not diagnostic) |
| Increase in peak velocity on serial studies (more reliable) |
| Impaired right ventricular function |

 **MISTAKES TO AVOID**

- Using the tricuspid regurgitant jet to estimate pulmonary artery systolic pressure with a pulmonary valve replacement in situ

**CHECKLIST FOR REPORTING TRICUSPID OR PULMONARY VALVES**

1. Appearance of the valve
2. $V_{max}$ and mean gradient (both positions) and pressure half-time (tricuspid)
3. Presence, location and grade of regurgitation
4. RV size and function:
   a. Dilated and hyperdynamic with severe tricuspid or pulmonary regurgitation
   b. Small in severe tricuspid stenosis
   c. Dilated and hypokinetic in pulmonary stenosis
5. Size of pulmonary artery

# References

1. Jamieson WR. Update on technologies for cardiac valvular replacement, and transcatheter innovations, and reconstructive surgery. 2010;20:255–81.
2. Zoghbi WA, Chambers JB, Dumesnil JG et al. American Society of Echocardiography recommendations for evaluation of prosthetic valves with two-dimensional and Doppler echocardiography. *J Am Soc Echocardiogr* 2009;22:975–1014.
3. Grunkemeier GL, Li H-H, Naftel DC, Starr A, Rahimtoola SH. Long-term performance of heart valve prostheses. *Curr Prob Cardiol* 2000;25:73–156
4. Nishimura RA, Otto CM, Bonow RO et al. 2014 AHA/ACC guideline for the management of patients with valvular heart disease. *J Am Coll Cardiol* 2014;63:e57–e185.
5. Zamorano JL, Badano LP, Bruce C et al. EAE/ASE recommendations for the use of echocardiography in new transcatheter interventions for valvular heart disease. *J Am Soc Echocardiogr* 2011;24:937–65 and *Eur Heart J* 2011;32:2189–214.
6. Connolly HM, Miller FA, Jr., Taylor CL, Naessens JM, Seward JB, Tajik AJ. Doppler hemodynamic profiles of 82 clinically and echocardiographically normal tricuspid valve prostheses. *Circulation* 1993;88(6):2722–7.
7. Kobayashi Y, Nagata S, Ohmori F, Eishi K, Nakano K, Miyatake K. Serial doppler echocardiographic evaluation of bioprosthetic valves in the tricuspid position. *J Am Coll Cardiol* 1996;27(7):1693–7.
8. Novaro GM, Connolly HM, Miller FA. Doppler hemodynamics of 51 clinically and echocardiographically normal pulmonary valve prostheses. *Mayo Clinic Proceedings* 2001;76(2):155–60.

# Endocarditis

## 11

Infective endocarditis is uncommon (up to 10 cases per 100,000 population per year) but the mortality is high at 20%, and about 40% need inpatient cardiac surgery.[1] The diagnosis is aided by the Duke criteria (Appendix 3: Table A3.3) which include vegetation, local complication or valve destruction on the echocardiogram as major criteria.

## 1 Is there a vegetation?

- This is typically a mass attached to the valve and moving with a different phase to the leaflet. It may sometimes be integral to the leaflet.
- It may be difficult to differentiate from other types of masses (e.g. calcific or myomatous degeneration, a fibrin strand or flail chord). This is a particular problem if echocardiography has been requested with a low clinical likelihood of endocarditis. Choose a descriptive term that will not lead to overdiagnosis of endocarditis (Table 11.1).
- Note the size and mobility of the vegetation. Highly mobile masses larger than 10 mm in length[2] have a relatively high risk of embolisation and may affect the decision for surgery.
- Vegetations usually occur on valves but also at the site of jet lesions or around the orifice of a VSD.

**Table 11.1** Suggested terms for describing a mass

| |
| --- |
| 'typical of a vegetation' |
| 'consistent with a vegetation' |
| 'consistent but not diagnostic of a vegetation' |
| 'consistent with a vegetation but more in keeping with calcific degeneration' |
| 'most consistent with calcific degeneration' |

**INK!**

## 2 Is there a local complication?

- A new paraprosthetic leak is a reliable sign of prosthetic endocarditis provided there is a baseline postoperative study showing no leak.
- An abscess usually suggests that surgery will be necessary.
- TTE is good for showing anterior root abscesses (Figure 11.1); TOE is better for posterior root abscesses.

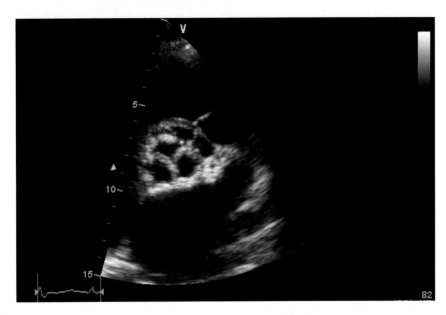

Figure 11.1 Aortic abscess. Parasternal short-axis view showing cavities between the pulmonary artery and aorta and in the anterior aorta. The aortic valve cusps are thickened because of endocarditis.

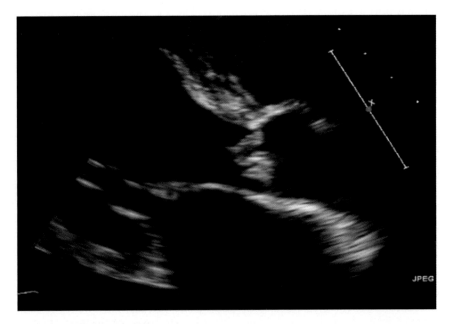

Figure 11.2 Valve destruction.

# 3 Is there valve destruction?

- This may show as:
  - disruption of the leaflet tissue with unusual patterns of movement, 'dog-legs' or small flail segments (Figure 11.2)
  - a perforation
  - new prolapse
  - new or worsening regurgitation.

# 4 Check the other valves

- Multiple valve involvement is particularly likely with invasive organisms, e.g. *Staphylococcus aureus.*
- The jet of aortic regurgitation may impinge on the anterior mitral leaflet to seed a vegetation or cause local infection leading to an aneurysm or perforation.

# 5 Assess the grade of regurgitation

- This is as for regurgitation from any cause (Chapters 7–9).
- The colour jet and spectral Doppler may be difficult to interpret because of artefact caused by the vibration of a vegetation, ruptured chord or torn leaflet (Figure 11.3). A hyperdynamic LV is a clue to severity.
- The presence of severe regurgitation informs the timing of surgery, especially if there is LV dysfunction.

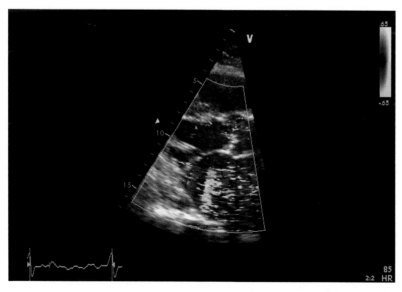

**Figure 11.3 Comb artefact.** This is caused by the vibration of a vegetation attached to the posterior mitral leaflet and leads to colour filling the left atrium and extending outside the heart.

And here's an electronic link to a loop on the website or use
http://goo.gl/0kP3od

## 6 Assess the LV

● Progressive systolic dilatation of the LV aids the decision for surgery.
● If there is acute severe aortic regurgitation, look for a transmitral E deceleration time <150 ms on pulsed Doppler. This is a sign of a raised LV end-diastolic pressure and an indication for urgent surgery.

## 7 Detect a predisposing abnormality

● About one half of cases develop on previously normal valves, but predisposing abnormalities are given in Table 11.2.
● Pacemaker and implantable defibrillator endocarditis is increasingly common.

Table 11.2 Predisposing abnormalities

| |
|---|
| Native heart valve disease |
| Replacement heart valves |
| Prior endocarditis |
| Congenital disease (other than ASD)[3] |
| Hypertrophic cardiomyopathy |
| Implantable pacemaker or defibrillator |

## 8 TTE is normal despite a clinical suspicion of endocarditis

● This requires clinical discussion and depends on the clinical likelihood of endocarditis, how ill the patient is and the quality of the transthoracic images.
● If the clinical likelihood is low or an alternative diagnosis emerges, echocardiography is not indicated.
● If the clinical likelihood is moderate or high, choices include immediate TOE or a further TTE ± TOE after 7–10 days.[4, 5]

## 9 When is TOE necessary?

● Established indications are given in Table 11.3.
● TOE is commonly necessary if there is a prosthetic valve or pacemaker or defibrillator because the yield of vegetations and complications is higher.

- Guidelines[6, 7] suggest a low threshold for requesting TOE even if the diagnosis has been established by TTE with the rationale that it will refine the assessment of vegetation size and exclude complications. In clinical practice TOE is not usually necessary if the results would not change management (e.g. decision for surgery already made).

**Table 11.3** Indications for TOE in endocarditis

| |
|---|
| Replacement heart valve especially mechanical if diagnosis not established |
| Pacemaker or implantable defibrillator |
| Suspicion of abscess on transthoracic study or clinically (e.g. long PR interval) |
| Normal or equivocal transthoracic study and moderate or high clinical suspicion of endocarditis |

 **MISTAKES TO AVOID**

- Echocardiography should not be used as part of a fever screen since it then has a very low yield and risks detecting 'innocent bystander' abnormalities (e.g. coincidental aortic valve thickening)
- Reporting innocent bystander findings as vegetations
- Missing progressive valve regurgitation as a sign of endocarditis
- Overusing TOE when it will not change management

**CHECKLIST FOR REPORTING ENDOCARDITIS**

1. Is there a vegetation, local complication or evidence of valve destruction?
2. Grade of regurgitation?
3. Presence and severity of predisposing disease (e.g. valve stenosis or VSD)
4. LV dimensions and function (or RV for tricuspid valve endocarditis)
5. Is there a restrictive filling pattern as evidence of high LV filling pressures?

# References

1. Chambers J, Sandoe J, Ray S et al. The infective endocarditis team: recommendations from an international working group. *Heart* 2014;100:524–7.
2. Thuny F, Disalvo G, Belliard O et al. Risk of embolism and death in infective endocarditis: prognostic value of echocardiography: a prospective multicenter study. *Circulation* 2005;112:69–75.
3. Verheugt CL, Uiterwaal CSPM, van der Velde ET, et al. Turning 18 with congenital heart disease: prediction of infective endocarditis based on a very large population. *Eur Heart J* 2011;32:1926–34.
4. Vieira MLC, Grinberg M, Pomerantzeff PMA, Andrade JL, Mansur AJ. Repeated echocardiographic examinations of patients with suspected infective endocarditis. *Heart* 2004;90:1020.
5. Habib G, Badano L, Tribouilloy C et al. Recommendations for the practice or echocardiography in infective endocarditis. *Eur J Echocardiogr* 2010;11:202–19.
6. Baddour LM., Wilson WR, Bayer AS et al. Infective endocarditis: diagnosis, antimicrobial therapy, and management of complications: a statement for healthcare professionals from the Committee on Rheumatic Fever, Endocarditis, and Kawasaki Disease, Council on Cardiovascular Disease in the Young, and the Councils on Clinical Cardiology, Stroke, and Cardiovascular Surgery and Anesthesia, American Heart Association – executive summary: endorsed by the Infectious Diseases Society of America. *Circulation* 2005;111:3394–434.
7. Habib G, Hoen B, Tornos P et al. Guidelines on the prevention, diagnosis, and treatment of infective endocarditis (new version 2009). *Eur Heart J* 2009;30:2369–413.

## The aorta

- The root refers to the aorta between the annulus and the sinotubular junction (Figure 12.1). The diameter of the sinus of valsalva is measured as part of the minimum standard study.
- Above this, the ascending aorta extends from the sinotubular junction to the arch and may be less easily imaged than the root. Additional windows (suprasternal

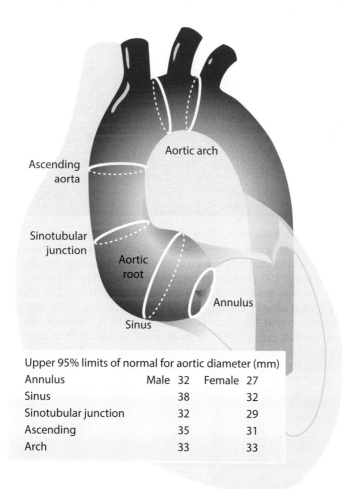

| Upper 95% limits of normal for aortic diameter (mm) | | |
| --- | --- | --- |
| Annulus | Male 32 | Female 27 |
| Sinus | 38 | 32 |
| Sinotubular junction | 32 | 29 |
| Ascending | 35 | 31 |
| Arch | 33 | 33 |

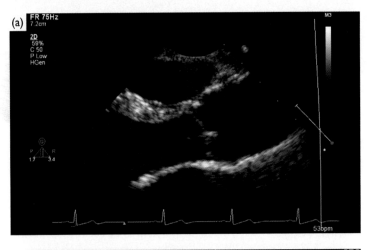

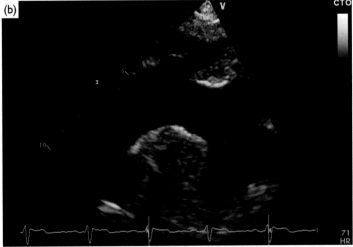

**Figure 12.1 Levels for measuring the diameter of the aorta.** The thoracic aorta is divided into: (1) the root between the annulus and the top of the sinuses; (2) the ascending aorta between the sinotubular junction and the start of the innominate artery; (3) the arch between the innominate artery and 2 cm beyond the left sublavian artery; (4) the descending thoracic aorta from the isthmus 2 cm beyond the left sublavian artery and the diaphragm. The upper abdominal aorta around the level of the celiac axis is imaged from subcostal views. (a) Representative parasternal long-axis view of the aorta for measuring diameters at the annulus, sinus sinotubular junction and ascending aorta. (b) Suprasternal view for measuring the arch diameter.

notch, right intercostal spaces and high left parasternal views) are necessary if there is a high likelihood of dilatation, for example:

- dilatation of the root or ascending aorta on the initial views
- significant aortic valve disease (stenosis or regurgitation)
- bicuspid aortic valve
- congenital syndromes associated with aortic dilatation, e.g. Marfan syndrome (Table 12.1).

**Table 12.1** Causes of aortic dilatation

| |
|---|
| Atherosclerosis (hypertension, smoking, age) |
| Congenital syndromes: Marfan Syndrome, Ehlers–Danlos Type IV, Loeys–Dietz, Turner's |
| Annuloaortic ectasia |
| Bicuspid valve |
| Infections – syphilis, *Staphylococcus aureus* |
| Inflammatory diseases – Takayasu, giant cell arteritis, Behçet's syndrome, rheumatoid arthritis, ankylosing spondylitis |
| Trauma* – deceleration injury, cardiac catheterisation |
| Dissection* |

*These usually present acutely but occasionally chronically

- There is no international consensus on how to measure the diameters other than to use 2D rather than M-mode:
  - 'Inner to inner' rather than 'leading edge to leading edge' is recommended in more recent guidelines.[1, 2] This is concordant with CT and CMR.
  - Many normal ranges use diastole, but the 'largest diameter obtainable' is also recommended.[3]
  - We suggest that individual laboratories agree a standard (e.g. inner to inner on the clearest image obtainable, usually in diastole).
  - If thresholds for surgery are close, it is usual to confirm aortic size using CT or CMR.
- Upper 95% limits for normal based on multiple imaging modalities are given in Table 12.2. Guideline thresholds for abnormal dilatation are:
  - ascending aorta >40 mm (>21 mm/m$^2$).
  - descending aorta >35 mm (>16 mm/m$^2$)
  - abdominal >30 mm.
- However, aortic size is related to body habitus and age. Graphs are shown in Appendix 5 for BSA (Figure A5.1), height (Figure A5.2) and age (Figure A5.3).
- The shape may give a guide. Annuloaortic ectasia causes a pear-shaped root.
- A difference in proportion can be used to diagnose dilatation, e.g. an ascending: descending thoracic aorta diameter >1.5. The diameter of the ascending aorta and sinotubular junction should be similar and slightly larger than the annulus.
- The site of dilatation varies with the cause:[4]
  - Marfan syndrome: typically 'pear-shaped' annuloaortic ectasia
  - bicuspid valve: ascending aorta more than sinus
  - atherosclerosis (degenerative): sinus and ascending aorta.

- If the ascending aorta cannot be imaged adequately, use CMR or CT.
- Minimum thresholds for referral for surgery are given (Table 12.3) although the timing of surgery takes account of many clinical factors and must be individualised.

**Table 12.2** Suggested upper 95% limits of normal for aortic diameter (mm) measure leading edge (LE) or inner to inner (Inner) in diastole

| Site | Male | | Female | | Ref |
|---|---|---|---|---|---|
| | Upper limit | Indexed | Upper limit | Indexed | |
| Annulus (LE) | 32 | 15 | 27 | 15 | 6 |
| Sinus (Inner) | 38 | 19 | 32 | 20 | 7 |
| Sinus (LE) | 41 | 21 | 35 | 22 | 7 |
| STJ (Inner) | 32 | 20 | 29 | 18 | 7 |
| STJ (LE) | 37 | 19 | 31 | 20 | 7 |
| Ascending (Inner) | 35 | 18 | 31 | 19 | 7 |
| Ascending (LE) | 36 | 19 | 32 | 20 | 7 |
| Arch | 33 | | 33 | | 8 |
| Descending | 31 | 16 | 28 | 16 | 9* 10† |
| Abdominal (high) | 27 | | 23 | | 11* |

LE: leading edge; STJ: sinotubular junction
*CT
†TOE

**Table 12.3** Guideline thresholds for surgical referral in aortic dilatation[1, 11, 12]

| Ascending thoracic aorta | |
|---|---|
| Atherosclerotic dilatation or bicuspid aortic valve | 55 mm[13]* |
| Marfan | 50 mm[13, 14] |
| Bicuspid valve + risk factors† | 50 mm (or 25 mm/m[2])[12] |
| Marfan + risk factors† | 45 mm[1] |
| **Isolated arch** | 55 mm[1] |

| Descending thoracic or upper abdominal ('thoracoabdominal') | |
|---|---|
| Post dissection | 55 mm[1] |
| Degenerative or saccular and stenting feasible | 55 mm[1] |
| Degenerative or saccular and stenting not possible | 60 mm[1] |

The maximum diameter is used regardless of level
*Or >27.5 mm/m$^2$ in patients with small BSA, e.g. Turner's syndrome
[†]risk factors: high rate of increase (e.g. >3 mm/yr), Family history of dissection, uncontrolled hypertension, coarctation

## Other features

- **Is the aortic wall thickened?** (≥5 mm)
- **Is there significant calcification in the aorta?** Severe calcification may affect the feasibility of surgery.
- **How much aortic regurgitation?** See Table 7.8, page 71.
- **Has the aortic diameter changed from previous studies?** A significant increase is taken as >3 mm in one year.[12] Check by comparing the images that the measurements were taken from at the same level and in the same part of the cycle.
- **How long is the abnormal part of the aorta?** If the ascending aorta is dilated, check whether the arch and descending thoracic aorta are normal. This may require imaging using CT or CMR if echo image quality is not adequate.
- **Check for coarctation** in all subjects, particularly if there is a bicuspid aortic valve or unexplained aortic dilatation in a young subject.
- **Is there mitral or tricuspid prolapse?** This is relevant in patients with Marfan syndrome or Ehlers–Danlos.
- **Is there coexistent pulmonary artery dilatation?** See Table 9.7. This may be seen in Marfan syndrome and to a lesser degree with bicuspid aortic valve.
- **Consider measuring the descending thoracic and abdominal aorta**. Use all views (parasternal long-axis both standard and rotated to show the aorta longitudinally, suprasternal, subcostal and abdominal). This should be done in:
  - Marfan syndrome and Ehlers–Danlos
  - dissection
  - dilatation of the arch
  - dilatation of the descending aorta shown on initial parasternal long-axis view.

# Dissection

- Acute aortic syndrome refers to the presentation with instantaneous onset chest pain often in patients with an underlying predisposition (e.g. Marfan syndrome, known aortic valve or aortic disease) and suggestive clinical findings (asymmetric pulses or blood pressure).
- The main cause is dissection for which TTE is useful. This affects the ascending aorta (Type A) or the descending aorta alone (Type B) (Figure 12.2).
- TOE, CT or CMR are needed to detect the other causes: intramural haematoma (20% acute aortic syndromes); penetrating ulcer (5% of acute aortic syndromes); aortic pseudoaneurysms, and contained or free rupture (usually after trauma or surgery).

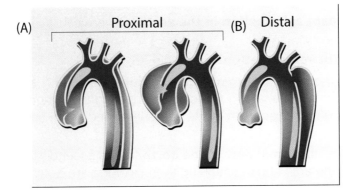

**Figure 12.2 Classification of dissections.** Type A dissections involve the ascending aorta. Type B dissections involve only the descending thoracic aorta.

## 1 Is there a dissection flap?

- An intraluminal flap is the hallmark of dissection. Blooming from calcium deposits or reverberation artefact can sometimes cause confusion. Factors suggesting artefact:
  - Fixed relationship with a heavy reflector e.g. anterior aortic wall
  - No movement at a phase different from the aorta
  - Only apparent in certain views
  - 'Pseudoflap' extends outside the aorta
  - The 'pseudoflap' has no effect on colour Doppler (a real flap would divide colour onto true and false lumens or there would be increased velocities through entry tears)
- Transthoracic echocardiography has 80% sensitivity for ascending aortic dissections and 50–70% for descending aortic dissections. This is increased using transpulmonary contrast.[15]

- If the study appears normal:
  - Check all views obtainable including suprasternal and right intercostal.
  - Consider intramural haematoma. Check for thickening of the aortic wall (>5 mm).
  - CT or TOE (Table 12.4) is always necessary if the clinical suspicion of dissection is high even when the TTE is normal.
- Even if TOE is needed to delineate an intrathoracic flap, TTE is better at showing the distal extent of the dissection in the abdominal aorta.

**Table 12.4** Role of TOE in suspected dissection

| |
| --- |
| Detection of dissection flap |
| Detection of mural haematoma |
| Aortic diameters |
| Entry tear |
| Involvement of head and neck vessels |
| Thrombosis of the false lumen |

## 2 What is the maximum aortic diameter?

Dissection is unlikely in an aorta of normal diameter.

## 3 How much aortic regurgitation is there?

See Table 7.8, page 71.

## 4 Is there pericardial fluid?

This suggests rupture into the pericardial sac, which is a common cause of death in acute dissection. It may suggest the diagnosis even if a flap cannot be imaged.

## 5 LV function

Impaired LV function on TTE can guide the decision for conservative management especially in dissections involving only the descending thoracic aorta.

## 6 Other techniques

- CT and CMR can be used to image parts of the aorta not accessible to echocardiography and are usually recommended if the aortic diameter on TTE is close to a threshold for surgery.
- CT may be used to detect aortic dissection or other cause of acute aortic syndromes if the TTE and clinical setting are inconclusive.

**MISTAKES TO AVOID**

- Making oblique measurements of the aortic diameter, particularly in off-axis views
- Overdiagnosis of dissection from a reverberation artefact
- Failing to image the ascending aorta when clinically necessary
- Monitoring aortic size using echocardiography alone if image quality is not adequate

## CHECKLIST FOR REPORTING THE AORTA

1. Diameter at each level. Have any changed?
2. Aortic regurgitation
3. If there is Marfan syndrome:
   a. Mitral and tricuspid prolapse and annular calcification
   b. Pulmonary artery diameter
4. If there is suspected dissection (see page 156):
   a. Is there a flap?
   b. Is there a pericardial effusion?
5. If there is a coarctation:
   a. Site
   b. Peak systolic velocity and presence of diastolic forward flow
   c. Aortic diameter above and below the coarctation and in the ascending aorta
   d. Check for bicuspid aortic valve and associated LV hypertrophy

## References

1. Hiratzka LF, Bakris GL, Beckman JA et al. Guidelines for the diagnosis and management of patients with thoracic aortic disease. *J Am Coll Cardiol* 2010;55:e27–129.
2. Evangelista A, Flachskampf FA, Erbel R et al. Echocardiography in aortic diseases: EAE recommendations for clinical practice. *Eur J Echocardiogr* 2010;11:645–58.
3. Lang RM, Bierig M, Devereux RB et al. Recommendations for chamber quantification. *Eur J Echocardiogr* 7(2):79–108, 2006.
4. Detain D et al. Aortic dilatation patterns and rates in adults with bicuspid aortic valves: a comparative study with Marfan syndrome and degenerative aortopathy. *Heart* 2014;100: 126–34.

5.  Roman MJ, Devereux RB, Kramer-Fox R, O'Loughlin J. Two-dimensional echocardiographic aortic root dimensions in normal children and adults. *Am J Cardiol* 1989;64:507–12.

6.  Muraru D, Maffessanti F, Kocabay G et al. Ascending aorta diameters measured by echocardiography using both leading edge-to-leading edge and inner edge-to-inner edge conventions in healthy volunteers. *Eur Heart J – Cardiovasc Imaging* 2014;15:415–22.

7.  Triulzi MO, Gillam LD, Gentile F. Normal adult cross-sectional echocardiographic values: linear dimensions and chamber areas. *Echocardiography* 1984;1:403–26.

8.  Wolak A, Gransar H, Thomson LEJ et al. Aortic size assessment by noncontrast cardiac computed tomography: normal limits by age, gender, and body surface area.*JACC CI* 2008;1:200–9.

9.  Drexler M, Erbel R, Muller U, Wittlich N, Mohr-Kahaly S, Meyer J. Measurement of intracardiac dimensions and structures in normal young adult subjects by transesophageal echocardiography. *Am J Cardiol* 1990; 65:1491–6.

10. Rutherford RB et al. Suggested standards for reporting on arterial aneurysms. *J Vasc Surg* 1991;13:452–8.

11. Vahanian A, Alfieri O, Andreotti F et al. Guidelines on the management of valvular heart disease (version 2012). *Eur Heart J* 2012;33:2451–95.

12. Erbel R, Aboyans V, Boileau C et al. 2014 ESC guidelines on the diagnosis and treatment of aortic diseases. *Eur Heart J* 2014;35:2873–2926.

13. Elefteriades JA. Natural history of thoracic aortic aneurysms: indications for surgery, and surgical versus nonsurgical risks. *Ann Thorac Surg* 2002;74(5):S1877–80; discussion S1892–8.

14. Ergin MA, Spielvogel D, Apaydin A et al. Surgical treatment of the dilated ascending aorta: when and how? *Ann Thorac Surg* 1999;67(6):1834–9; discussion 1853–6.

15. Evangelista A, Avegliano G, Aguilar R et al. Impact of contrast-enhanced echocardiography on the diagnostic algorithm of acute aortic dissection. *Eur Heart J* 2010;31:472–9.

# The atria and atrial septum

# 13

## The left atrium

Left atrial (LA) geometry varies and is not accurately represented by a linear dimension. Left atrial size needs to be assessed more accurately if:

- atrial diameter >40 mm in the parasternal long-axis view
- hypertension (as a sign of chronically increased filling pressure)
- atrial fibrillation (likely success of cardioversion, thromboembolic risk)
- mitral valve disease (thromboembolic risk, indirect marker of severity)
- suspected LV diastolic heart failure.

  Note the following:

- **Diameter:** A single left atrial diameter measurement is still recorded in routine clinical practice using 2D usually in a parasternal long-axis view. Normal is <40 mm.
- **Area:** A simple clinical method is planimetry of the area in a 4-chamber view excluding the appendage and pulmonary veins. The view may be modified if necessary to optimise atrial size (Table 13.1) and frozen at maximum size just before mitral valve opening.
- **Volume:** Planimeter the area in the 4-chamber and 2-chamber views and index to BSA. Biplane Simpson's and area–length methods are both used but for serial assessments a consistent method should be used.
- If there is a left atrial mass, see Chapter 16.

Table 13.1 Grading left atrial size in males and females[1, 2]

|  | Normal | Mildly dilated | Moderately dilated | Severely dilated |
|---|---|---|---|---|
| LA area (cm²) | <20 | 20–30 | 31–40 | >40 |
| LA vol/BSA (ml/m²) | 16–34 | 35–41 | 42–48 | >48 |

## The right atrium

Right atrial (RA) size needs to be assessed more accurately if:

- it looks similar in size or larger than the LA in the 4-chamber view
- there is atrial fibrillation (likely success of cardioversion, thromboembolic risk)

- there is suspected right or left ventricular dysfunction
- there is pulmonary hypertension
- there is an ASD
- there is tricuspid valve disease.

The right atrium is measured at end systole in the apical 4-chamber view where a planimetered area >18 cm² or a transverse diameter of >44 mm indicates dilatation. Volume measurements are not currently recommended.[3]

- Atrial dilatation can give a clue to the diagnosis (Table 13.2).
- If there is a right atrial mass, see Chapter 16.

Table 13.2 Causes of atrial enlargement

| **Characteristically biatrial** |
| --- |
| Apical hypertrophic cardiomyopathy |
| Restrictive cardiomyopathy |
| Rheumatic disease affecting mitral and tricuspid valves |
| Chronic atrial fibrillation |
| Pericardial constriction (mild or moderate enlargement) |
| **Predominantly left-sided** |
| Mitral stenosis or regurgitation |
| Left ventricular diastolic dysfunction |
| **Predominantly right-sided** |
| Tricuspid stenosis or regurgitation (Chapter 9) |
| Pulmonary hypertension (Chapter 6) |
| ASD (Chapter 14) |
| RV myopathy |

# The atrial septum

## 1 Is the septum thickened?

- Lipomatous hypertrophy is normal and occurs in a dumb-bell shaped distribution sparing the fossa ovalis in the middle.
- An attached mass suggests a myxoma or less commonly a thrombus caught in a patent foramen ovale (PFO).

## 2 Is the septum mobile or aneurysmal?

- An atrial septal aneurysm is defined[4] (Figure 13.1) by:
  - a mobile segment with base >10 mm wide, and
  - excursion ≥10 mm between left and right atrium during spontaneous respiration.
- A mobile septum is defined by an excursion of <10 mm and has no pathological significance.
- An aneurysmal septum is often associated with a PFO. The presence of both together is associated with a significantly higher recurrence rate after cardioembolic stroke than with either alone.
- Bowing of the whole septum may also occur as a result of severe TR or MR or high RA or LA pressures, e.g. ventricular dysfunction.
- Sometimes the aneurysm is fixed.

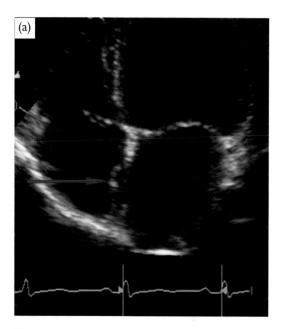 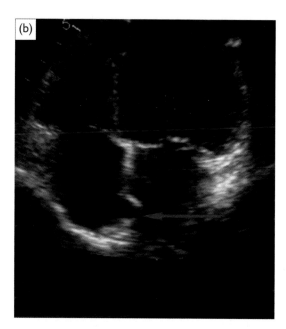

Figure 13.1 Atrial septal aneurysm. Maximum rightward (a) and leftward (b) extent.

## 3 ASD or dropout?

- In the 4-chamber view it is common to see dropout. The uncertainty is usually resolved on other views and by the absence of abnormal flow on colour mapping.

- If doubt still remains, consider:
  - a saline contrast injection which may make the ASD obvious as a void
  - pulsed Doppler on the right atrial side of the septum. ASD flow has a peak in late diastole and systole. For the superior vena cava, the peaks are earlier.
  - TOE or CMR.

## 4 Is there a PFO?

- These occur in 15% of the normal population[5] but may be more common:
  - after TIA or cerebral infarcts in young people
  - after decompression sickness in divers
  - in disproportionate hypoxia in critically ill patients
  - possibly in migraine with aura although this is not established.
- A PFO may be seen on colour imaging most frequently in a subcostal view.
- More usually, a bubble study is needed (Table 13.3). This is usually better performed transthoracically than on TOE.
- A PFO is usually taken to be present only if bubbles appear in the LA within three or fewer cardiac cycles after the injection.

- Grading a PFO is controversial:
  - Many thresholds for a large shunt appear in the literature (>10, >20, >25, >30 or >50 bubbles) although >20 has been most frequently used.
  - Counting individual bubbles is not usually easy in practice.
  - Imaging technology has improved recently making earlier thresholds in the literature outdated.
  - We use the system in Table 13.4.[6]
- Pulmonary capillary malformations are suggested by:
  - bubbles appearing after 3 cycles
  - early bubbles entering via the pulmonary veins
  - slow clearance of the bubbles as a result of continuing replenishment.

**Table 13.3 Performing a bubble contrast study**

| |
|---|
| 1. Allow adequate time. Practise the valsalva manoeuvre at the start ensuring that image quality is minimally affected and there is good leftward deviation of the atrial septum. |
| 2. Ask the patient to breathe out then hold the breath and strain with the abdomen against a closed glottis with minimal movement of the chest. Practise instant release. Place a 21 G cannula in an antecubital fossa vein and connect to a three-way tap. |

3. Fill a syringe with about 7–8 ml N saline. For each injection, leave approximately 0.5 ml air in the syringe and withdraw approximately 1 ml venous blood into the syringe. An alternative to saline is Gelofuscin and this is particularly useful if it is only possible to place a small peripheral cannula.
4. Attach a dry syringe to the other port of the 3-way tap and agitate between the two syringes until a dense froth containing no large air bubbles is produced.
5. For the initial injections there may be no manoeuvre. With the valsalva manoeuvre, the injection should be timed to reach the right heart at release. If the valsalva results are negative or equivocal, the patient can be asked to cough on right heart opacification.
6. A number of injections with valsalva should be given until attaining at least one with perfect synchronisation of all elements. Sometimes several (up to six) are necessary.
7. Archive about 8–10 cycles capturing the contrast arriving in the right heart and at least 5 cycles after this.

Table 13.4 Suggested method of grading a patent foramen ovale (Figure 13.2)

| Small | <20 bubbles |
|---|---|
| Moderate | More than about 20 bubbles, but not sufficient to cause a bolus within the left atrium or to fill the whole of the left heart (Figure 13.2a) |
| Large | Left atrial bolus of bubbles too numerous to count or bubbles filling the whole of the left heart (Figure 13.2b) |

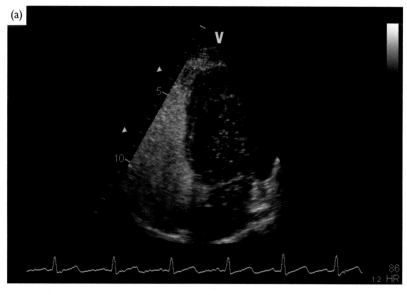

Figure 13.2a Bubble contrast study, moderate PFO.

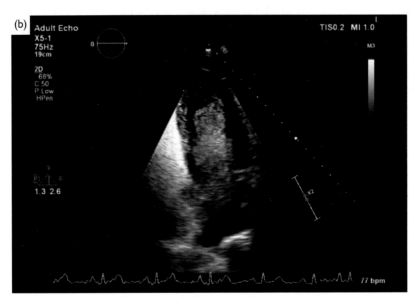

**Figure 13.2b  Bubble contrast study,** large PFO.

 MISTAKES TO AVOID

- Overdiagnosing atrial dilatation from a diameter in one plane
- Failing to coordinate a valsalva manoeuvre and the timing of the contrast injection when looking for a PFO
- Mistaking SVC flow for an ASD

## CHECKLIST FOR REPORTING THE ATRIA

1. Size of right and left atria
2. If dilated is there a cause (Table 13.2)?
3. Appearance of atrial septum
4. Is there evidence of a shunt?

# References

1. Lang RM, Bierig M, Devereux RB, Flachskampf FA, Foster E, Pellikka PA et al. Recommendations for chamber quantification. *Eur J Echocardiogr* 2006;7(2):79–108.
2. Lang RM, Badano LP, Mor-Avi V et al. Recommendations for cardiac chamber quantification by echocardiography in adults: an update from the American Society of Echocardiography and the European Association of Cardiovascular Imaging. *J Am Soc Echocardiogr* 2015;28:1–39.
3. Rudski L, Lai W, Afilalo J et al Guidelines for the echocardiographic assessment of the right heart in adults: a report from the American Society of Echocardiography. *J Am Soc Echocardiogr* 2010;23:685–713.
4. Mas JL, Arquizan C, Lamy C et al. Recurrent cerebrovascular events associated with patent foramen ovale, atrial septal aneurysm, or both. *N Engl J Med* 2001;345:1740–6.
5. Garg P, Servoss SJ, Wu JC, Bajwa ZH, Selim MH, Dineen A, Kuntz RE, Cook EF, Mauri L. Lack of association between migraine headache and patent foramen ovale. *Circulation* 2010;121:1404–12.
6. Chambers J, Seed P, Ridsdale L. Association of migraine aura with patent foramen ovale and atrial septal aneurysms. *Int J Cardiol* 2013;168:3949–53.

# Adult congenital disease | 14

- Patients with congenital disease are increasingly cared for at specialist centres, but they may still present as an emergency or be followed at a non-specialist centre with uncorrected simple lesions or after intervention.
- Examples of echocardiographic abnormalities found in congenital syndromes are given in Table 14.1.

**Table 14.1** Echocardiographic abnormalities in congenital syndromes

|  | Typical | Less common |
|---|---|---|
| Noonan | Dysplastic valvar pulmonary stenosis, HCM | ASD, VSD, branch PS, tetralogy of Fallot |
| Turner | Bicuspid AV, dilated aorta and coarctation |  |
| Williams | Supravalvar AS, coarctation | PA and branch stenosis |
| LEOPARD | Valvar PS, HCM |  |
| DiGeorge | Tetralogy of Fallot, VSD, truncus arteriosus | Interrupted arch |
| Alagille | Branch PS, tetralogy of Fallot | VSD, ASD, AS, coarctation |
| Keutel | Branch PS |  |
| Congenital rubella | Persistent duct, branch PS, coarctation |  |
| Foetal alcohol | VSD, ASD |  |
| Neurofibromatosis | Coarctation |  |
| Loeys–Dietz | Aortic dilatation | Bicuspid aortic valve, persistent ductus, ASD |

- A first diagnosis of a simple or occasionally a more complex lesion may still be made in a general echocardiography laboratory. This chapter describes:
  - simple defects
  - a systematic approach to an unexpected complex case
  - the appearances after intervention.
- Patients with congenital disease may be admitted acutely as a result of cardiac or other disease. Advice should be sought from a regional centre but findings of immediate concern include:
  - poorly functioning left or right ventricles

- severe valve obstruction or regurgitation
- evidence of endocarditis (the risk is 20 times higher than for the general population except for those with isolated pulmonary stenosis or ASD)[1]
- atrial arrhythmia (because of the risk of decompensation) in a Fontan circulation.

# Simple defects

## 1 Atrial septal defect (ASD)

See Table 14.2.

- This is the most common congenital defect found in adult practice.
- Think of the diagnosis if the right ventricle is dilated and active.
- Describe the position (Figure 14.1):
  - secundum (80% of ASDs) – approximately in the centre of the septum
  - primum (15% of ASD) – next to the atrioventricular valves (Table 14.3)
  - superior sinus venosus (5%) – may be difficult to image transthoracically; TOE or CMR is usually needed
  - rare: inferior sinus venosus and unroofed coronary sinus <1%.

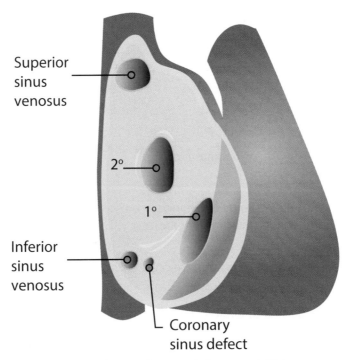

Superior sinus venosus

2°

1°

Inferior sinus venosus

Coronary sinus defect

Figure 14.1 Position of ASD. 1° is a primum defect and 2° is a secundum defect.

Table 14.2 Checklist in ASD

| Position (secundum, primum) |
| --- |
| Direction of shunt (left to right or bidirectional) |
| Anatomical and shunt size |
| RV size and function |
| PA pressure |
| LV size and function (may decompensate after ASD closure) |
| Other congenital or acquired defects? |

- Shunt direction? In adult practice this will usually be left to right, but if pulmonary vascular resistance is increased, flow may be right to left or bidirectional.
- Describe RV size and function (pages 47–50).
- Estimate pulmonary artery pressure (pages 53–54).
  - The systolic pressure may be elevated as a result of high right-sided flow.
  - If pulmonary resistance is not significantly raised, the diastolic pressure is normal or low.
  - Usually, if the PA systolic pressure is >50% systemic pressure, it is advisable to measure PA pressures and resistance invasively before considering closure.
- Estimate the anatomical and physiological size of the defect:
  - Secundum defect size can be measured approximately by callipers even on TTE but requires TOE for determining whether percutaneous closure is feasible.
  - RV dilatation (e.g. to the same cavity size in diastole as the normal LV) implies a haemodynamically significant shunt and is an indication for closure.
  - The shunt does not always need to be estimated (Appendix 4, section A4.8) since the decision for intervention is usually based on the presence of RV, page 228 volume load, but it may aid the initial diagnosis and help determine whether closure is still indicated if there is pulmonary hypertension.
- If there is a primum defect (Table 14.3), look for a ventricular inlet defect. Also assess the atrioventricular valves.
- TOE is indicated before device closure (Table 14.4) and TTE afterwards (Table 14.11).

Table 14.3 Features of a 'primum' ASD (part of the spectrum of atrioventricular septal defect)

| Defect adjacent to the atrioventricular valves |
| --- |
| Common atrioventricular valve rather than separate tricuspid and mitral valves:<br>• Lack of offset between left and right-sided atrioventricular valve<br>• Left atrioventricular valve appears 'cleft' or trileaflet |

(*continued*)

Table 14.3 Features of a 'primum' ASD (part of the spectrum of atrioventricular septal defect) (*continued*)

| Defect adjacent to the atrioventricular valves |
| --- |
| Long LV outflow tract caused by an offset between aortic valve and 'mitral valve' (normally the non-coronary aortic cusp is continuous with the base of the anterior mitral leaflet) |
| May be associated with a VSD |

Table 14.4 What to look for on TOE before device closure

| How many defects or fenestrations? |
| --- |
| Total septal length |
| • Diameter of defect and margins on imaging and colour in 4-chamber, aortic short-axis and bicaval views |
| Distance from atrioventricular valves |
| Distance from IVC and SVC |
| Distance from aorta (a margin is not necessary when an Amplatzer device is used) |
| Check correct drainage of pulmonary veins |
| Other defects especially cleft mitral valve |

- It is possible to mistake flow from the superior vena cava for flow across an ASD. Take multiple views. If there is still doubt, consider:
    - a saline contrast injection which may make the ASD obvious as a void
    - pulsed Doppler on the right atrial side of the septum: ASD flow has a peak in late diastole and systole; for the superior vena cava, the peaks are earlier
    - shunt calculation
    - TOE or CMR.

## 2 Ventricular septal defect

See Table 14.5.

- In the adult, a VSD may be newly diagnosed or unoperated as a child (either because it was too small or there was Eisenmenger syndrome) or it may be newly diagnosed.
- The possible late complications of a small VSD are:
    - increase in flow across the VSD as a result of increased LV pressures
    - jet lesion causing hypertrophy of the RV leading to a double-chambered RV
    - progressive aortic regurgitation caused by prolapse of the right or non-coronary aortic cusp (doubly committed, occasionally perimembranous VSD)
    - discrete subaortic stenosis.

- Localise the site of the defect (Figure 14.2):
  - perimembranous (80% of VSD)
  - muscular (15–20% of VSD) – these may be multiple
  - doubly committed (5% of VSD) – this may be associated with prolapse of the right or non-coronary cusp of the aortic valve. In a parasternal short-axis view it is adjacent to the pulmonary valve while a perimembranous defect is adjacent to the tricuspid valve
  - inlet
  - AVSD (see above).

Table 14.5 Checklist in VSD

| Position |
| --- |
| Size (anatomical and physiological) |
| Direction of shunt |
| LV size and evidence of overload |
| PA pressure |
| Other congenital or acquired defects |

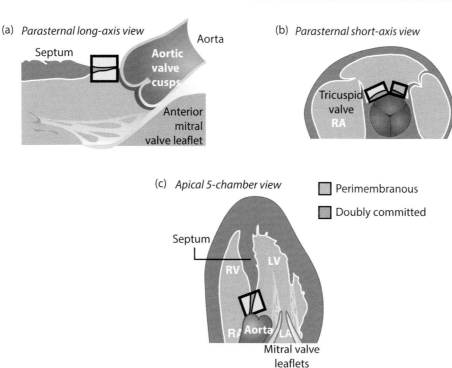

Figure 14.2 **Position of ventricular septal defects.** (a) Parasternal long-axis view; (b) parasternal short-axis view at aortic level; (c) apical 5-chamber view.

- Occasionally, muscular defects near the apex may be difficult to image but may first be detected using a stand-alone continuous wave probe placed where the murmur is most easily heard.
- Which direction is the shunt? In adult practice this will usually be left to right, but if the pulmonary vascular resistance is high, flow may be right to left or bidirectional.
- Estimate the size:
  - A restrictive defect (LV pressure is significantly higher than RV pressure) is shown by a $V_{max}$ across the lesion on continuous wave >4.0 m/s.
  - The shunt size can be estimated (Appendix 4, Table A4.1) as a guide, but the LV size and activity are usually used as an indication for surgery in asymptomatic patients.
  - In the presence of pulmonary hypertension, a left-to-right shunt >1.5 and a PA systolic pressure (or pulmonary vascular resistance) <2/3 systemic levels indicates that surgery may still be considered.[2]
- Assess the left ventricle. Left ventricular volume load suggests a large shunt. Volume overload and systolic dilatation are criteria for closure.
- Assess the right ventricle. Hypertrophy of muscular bands may be associated with a perimembranous defect causing a double-chambered right ventricle.
- Estimate pulmonary artery pressures (pages 53–54).
  - Be careful to position the cursor away from VSD flow when recording TR $V_{max}$.
  - If the PA systolic pressure is >50% systemic pressure, it is usually advisable to measure PA pressures and resistance invasively before considering closure.

## 3 Persistent ductus

See Table 14.6. The persistent ductus arteriosus (PDA) is a channel between the descending thoracic aorta and the left pulmonary branch. It is usually at or beyond the left subclavian artery level.

Table 14.6 Checklist in persistent ductus arteriosus

| |
|---|
| Size |
| Direction of flow |
| LV size and function (volume load in moderate or large persistent ductus) |
| PA size (commonly dilated) |
| Pulmonary artery pressure |
| RV function (pressure load with Eisenmenger physiology) |
| Other defects? |

- Look for reversed flow in the main pulmonary artery using parasternal short- and long-axis views and for the defect in the suprasternal view (Figure 14.3a).
- Estimate pulmonary artery pressure (pages 53–54). When raised, flow through the duct may diminish, cease or reverse during systole. When normal, flow is continuous throughout the cardiac cycle (Figure 14.3b).
- Estimate the shunt size (Appendix 4, Table A4.1). LV volume-load suggests a large shunt.

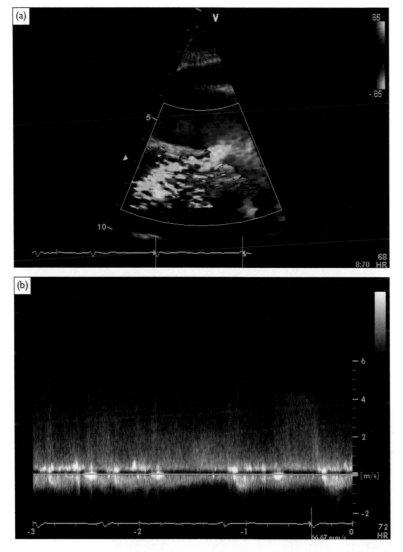

**Figure 14.3 Persistent ductus.** The defect from a suprasternal position (a) and on continuous wave (b) from a parasternal window in a large duct with normal pulmonary pressures.

# 4 Coarctation

See Table 14.7.

- Coarctation is a narrowing of the aorta, usually just beyond the left subclavian artery at the site of the ductus arteriosus. It is part of a generalised left-sided arteriopathy.
- Always check for this in patients with:
  - bicuspid aortic valve
  - early onset systemic hypertension
  - murmur
  - syndromes associated with coarctation (Turner, Williams, congenital rubella, neurofibromatosis).

## 4.1 Appearance

- Describe the site and appearance (membrane, tunnel) using imaging and colour flow.
- Measure aortic dimensions above and below the coarctation.
- Look for associated aortic root dilatation and bicuspid aortic valve.
- Check for LV hypertrophy and LV systolic and diastolic function.

## 4.2 Continuous wave Doppler

- The most reliable feature on continuous wave recording is forward flow during diastole (Figure 14.4). Elevated flow velocities are usually seen in systole, but may occasionally be absent or difficult to record if there is a severe or complete coarctation with extensive collaterals.
- Intervention is not decided by the velocities or gradients across the coarctation but by the presence of systemic hypertension and:
  - a pressure difference >20 mmHg between upper and lower limbs, or
  - narrowing ⩾50% relative to aortic diameter at diaphragm level on CT or CMR.

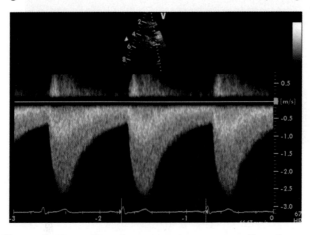

**Figure 14.4 Coarctation.** Continuous wave recording from the suprasternal notch.

Table 14.7 Checklist in coarctation

| Site |
| --- |
| Morphology (membrane, tunnel) |
| Systolic and diastolic flow |
| Presence of bicuspid valve |
| Diameter of aorta at all levels, ascending and descending thoracic and abdominal |
| LV adaptation especially hypertrophy |
| Other congenital or acquired defects |

## 5 Ebstein's anomaly

- This is characterised by:
  - apical displacement of the septal and posterior leaflets of the tricuspid valve towards the apex
  - division of the RV into an atrialised portion and a residual functional RV
  - usually tricuspid regurgitation.
- The diagnosis is often suspected from a combination of right-sided dilatation in the parasternal views and tricuspid regurgitation originating more apically than normal on the apical 4-chamber view.
- The haemodynamic effect of the anomaly is related to:
  - the size and function of the residual RV
  - the degree of tricuspid regurgitation
  - the presence of other congenital defects, especially ASD which occurs in about one-third.
- The echocardiographic checklist is in Table 14.8.
- Surgery is indicated[2, 3] for:
  - symptoms and more than moderate TR
  - progressive right-sided dilatation or reduction in right-sided function
  - systemic embolisation, when isolated closure of ASD or PFO may be indicated.

Table 14.8 Checklist in Ebstein's anomaly

| How much apical displacement of the septal and posterior leaflets (by definition >8 mm/m$^2$)? |
| --- |
| An elongated anterior leaflet meets the septal leaflet. How much tethering to the free wall? (Affects ability to repair the valve) |
| How much tricuspid regurgitation? |
| How large is the residual RV? (If greater than one-third of the total, makes repair more likely) |

(continued)

**Table 14.8** Checklist in Ebstein's anomaly (*continued*)

| Function of the residual RV |
| --- |
| Are there associated congenital defects?<br>• ASD (in about one-third), congenitally corrected transposition, pulmonary outflow stenosis<br>• 10% have left-sided abnormalities: cor triatriatum, cleft mitral valve, parachute mitral valve, bicuspid aortic valve |

## 6 Congenitally corrected transposition of the great arteries

See Table 14.9.

- Uncorrected transposition means that the aorta arises from the right ventricle and the pulmonary artery from the left ventricle. Survival after closure of the arterial duct requires associated congenital defects or palliative procedures to allow mixing of blood.
- In congenitally corrected transposition, the right atrium connects to a morphological left ventricle and thence to the pulmonary artery while the left atrium connects to a morphological right ventricle and thence to the aorta. This may present in adulthood. The key is that the systemic circulation is supplied by the morphological right ventricle.
- In congenitally corrected transposition, the right ventricle is always dilated and hypertrophied in response to the systemic pressure. Secondary tricuspid regurgitation may worsen ventricular function and may be suitable for intervention.

**Table 14.9** Echo features of congenitally corrected transposition

| Pulmonary artery and aorta in parallel on parasternal long-axis view |
| --- |
| Both valves seen together in a parasternal short-axis view |
| Ventricles reversed (morphological RV connected to the LA) |
| Dilated and hypertrophied morphological RV invariable |
| Tricuspid regurgitation |
| Associated congenital defects (VSD, PS, malformations of the tricuspid valve, complete heart block) |

 **MISTAKES TO AVOID**

- Mistaking VSD flow on continuous wave Doppler for tricuspid regurgitation in calculating PA pressures
- Failing to assess LV volume-load with a VSD as an indication for surgery
- Forgetting to look for an ASD in a volume-loaded right ventricle

# Systematic study

- Congenital disease should be suspected if specific abnormalities are found (Table 14.10).
- You may have little or no background information (e.g. new diagnosis, emergency admission, details of corrective surgery not available).

Table 14.10 Findings suspicious of congenital disease

| |
|---|
| Dilated or hypertrophied right ventricle |
| Pulmonary hypertension |
| Lack of offsetting in the 4-chamber view (endocardial cushion defect) |
| Abnormal offsetting (corrected transposition of the great arteries) |
| Pulmonary artery and aorta seen in parallel or pulmonary and aortic valves seen in the same parasternal short-axis view (corrected transposition of the great arteries) |
| Hyperdynamic left ventricle without aortic or mitral regurgitation |
| Dilated coronary sinus (usually left-sided SVC) |

- Perform a systematic study allowing a specialist review if necessary
- 'Atrioventricular valve' refers to the tricuspid and mitral and 'semilunar valve' to the pulmonary and aortic. Thus 'left atrioventricular valve' makes no assumptions that this is truly the mitral valve.
- 'Anatomical left ventricle' means the ventricle on the left of the heart; 'morphological left ventricle' means the ventricle attached to the mitral valve.
- 'Discordant' means incorrect connections, e.g. left atrium attached to morphological right ventricle or aorta leading from morphological right ventricle.

## 1 Are the atria correctly positioned?

- The morphological left and right atria are distinguished by their appendages, which may not be seen transthoracically, and the veins draining into them.
- Are the IVC and abdominal aorta normally related in an abdominal short-axis view? The aorta lies to the left of the spine and the IVC to the right.
- Follow the IVC (and SVC if visible) to the right atrium using subcostal views and check that this is on the correct side of the heart.

## 2 Are the atria attached to the correct ventricles?

- This is usually appreciated best from the apical 4-chamber view.
- The morphological right ventricle is recognised because:
  - its atrioventricular valve is more apical than the left-sided atrioventricular valve

- there is a gap between the atrioventricular valve and the semilunar valve
- there are more trabeculations than in the morphological left ventricle
- there is usually a moderator band.

## 3 Are the ventricles attached to the correct great arteries?

- The pulmonary artery bifurcates early and the aorta has an arch giving off the head and neck branch arteries.
- Congenitally corrected transposition of the great arteries is suspected if both great vessels can be imaged in transverse section from a parasternal short-axis view or longitudinally in a subcostal view.

## 4 Assess the size and systolic function of both ventricles

See pages 7–15 (LV) and 47–50 (RV).
- It is usual for a morphological right ventricle connected to the systemic circulation to be dilated and hypertrophied.

## 5 Estimate pulmonary artery pressure

See pages 53–54.
- Make sure to assess the atrioventricular valve jet from the ventricle connected to the pulmonary circulation.
- If there is outflow obstruction from valve stenosis or a band, the calculated pressures will reflect ventricular and not pulmonary artery systolic pressure.

## 6 Are there any shunts at atrial or ventricular level?

- Measure the size anatomically and estimate the shunt (Table A4.8, page 228).

## 7 Are the cardiac valves normal in appearance?

- Assess stenosis and regurgitation as for acquired valve disease.
- If there is no offsetting of the atrioventricular valves, the diagnosis is likely to be atrioventricular septal defect (Figure 14.5).

## 8 Is there aortic coarctation or a persistent duct?

See pages 156–157 (coarctation) and 154–155 (pda).

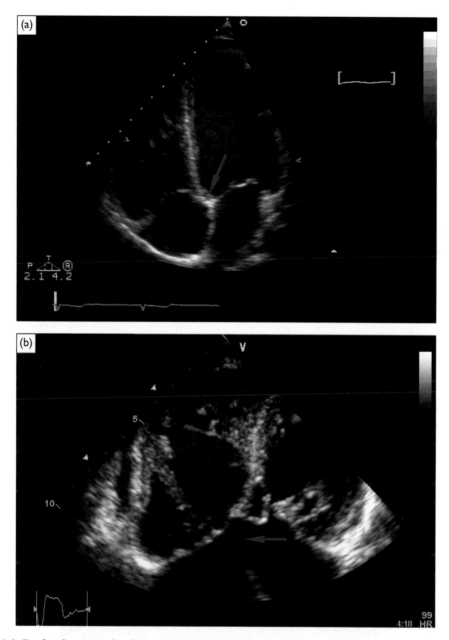

**Figure 14.5 Atrioventricular septal defect.** (a) A normal 4-chamber view showing that the tricuspid valve is offset (arrrow) or closer to the apex than the mitral valve. In (b) there is lack of offsetting, implying that there is a common AV valve. In addition, there is a large atrial septal defect (arrow).

## 9 Are the origins of the coronary arteries correctly positioned?

- In the parasternal short-axis view, the left coronary is usually seen at about 4 o'clock and the right at about 11 o'clock.

## 10 Is the coronary sinus dilated?

● This is usually caused by a left-sided SVC (image from the medial edge of the left supraclavicular fossa), occasionally by insertion of an aberrant coronary artery.

# Post-procedure studies

## 1 Device closure for an ASD or patent foramen ovale

See Table 14.11 and Figure 14.6.

● It is recommended[2, 3] that patients with residual shunts, raised PA pressure or who have been repaired late are followed at a specialist centre.

**Table 14.11** TTE checklist after device closure of an ASD or patent foramen ovale

| |
|---|
| Position of device |
| Is there any residual atrial shunt? Small leaks through or around the device (depending on the design) are normal and will disappear with time |
| Does the device obstruct the IVC or SVC? |
| Is the device close to the mitral valve and is there new or worse mitral regurgitation? |
| RV size and function (size may start to fall soon after closure) |
| Pericardial effusion (as a sign of perforation during the procedure) |
| PA pressure |
| LV size and systolic function |

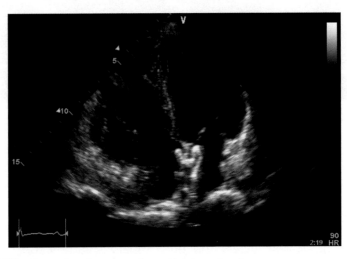

**Figure 14.6  ASD closed using an Amplatzer device.**

## 2 Closure of a VSD

See Table 14.12.

- After device closure, follow-up every 2–4 years beyond the first 2 years is recommended.[2, 3]

**Table 14.12** TTE checklist after closure of a VSD

| |
|---|
| Is there a residual shunt? |
| LV size and function |
| Aortic regurgitation if closure of perimembranous VSD |
| Pulmonary artery pressure |
| TR if surgical closure |
| (Check for complete heart block if device closure of perimembranous VSD) |

## 3 Closure of a persistent ductus

See Table 14.13.

- Patients with no residual shunt, normal LV and normal PA pressure do not need follow-up beyond 6 months.
- Patients with LV dysfunction or residual PA hypertension need follow-up at a specialist centre.

**Table 14.13** TTE checklist after closure of a persistent ductus

| |
|---|
| Is there a residual shunt? |
| LV size and function |
| Pulmonary artery pressure |
| Associated lesions |

## 4 Coarctation

See Table 14.14.

- Long-term follow-up is necessary.[2, 3]

**Table 14.14** TTE checklist after coarctation repair or stenting

| |
|---|
| Is there a residual, new or in-stent stenosis on imaging? |
| On continuous wave, an elevated systolic velocity is normal but there should be no diastolic forward flow |

(continued)

**Table 14.14** TTE checklist after coarctation repair or stenting (*continued*)

| |
|---|
| Assess the aorta beyond the repair looking for aneurysmal dilatation* |
| Assess the ascending aorta (which may be dilated) and aortic valve (may be bicuspid) |
| Assess LV size, function and hypertrophy |
| *Better performed with CMR |

# 5 Tetralogy of Fallot

See Table 14.15.

- Tetralogy of Fallot is caused by deviation of the outlet septum causing:
  - over-riding aorta
  - non-restrictive VSD
  - RV outflow obstruction (valvar or infundibular or both)
  - RV hypertrophy.
- The possible complications on echocardiography after repair are:
  - residual pulmonary regurgitation (especially if transannular PV patching was used)
  - residual RV outflow tract obstruction
  - residual branch PA stenosis if previous Blalock–Taussig shunt
  - RV dilatation caused by pulmonary regurgitation or stenosis and exacerbated by functional tricuspid regurgitation
  - residual VSD
  - aortic dilatation and resulting aortic regurgitation
  - LV dysfunction (due to cyanosis before repair or large VSD patch).

**Table 14.15** TTE checklist after repair of tetralogy of Fallot[4]

| |
|---|
| Position of agria |
| RV size and function including RV pressure |
| TR degree and mechanism:<br>• Patch disrupting septal-anterior commissure<br>• Annular dilatation<br>• Organic abnormality of the valve<br>• Pacing electrode |
| RA size |
| Is the VSD patch fully competent? |
| Assess pulmonary valve for stenosis and regurgitation |
| Assess branch pulmonary artery flow on colour and pulsed Doppler if possible |

| |
|---|
| Assess the RV outflow tract for muscular hypertrophy and/or aneurysm |
| LV size and function |
| Size of aortic root and ascending aorta and sidedness of aortic arch |
| Origin of coronary arteries |
| Degree of aortic regurgitation |
| Presence of systemic-to-pulmonary collateral vessels |
| Presence of associated anomalies |

## References

1. Verheugt CL, Uiterwaal CSPM, van der Velde ET et al. Turning 18 with congenital heart disease: prediction of infective endocarditis based on a very large population. *Eur Heart J* 2014;32:1926–34.
2. Baumgartner H, Bonhoeffer P, De Groot NMS et al. ESC guidelines for the management of grown-up congenital heart disease: The Task Force on the Management of Grown-up Congenital Heart Disease of the European Society of Cardiology (ESC). *Eur Heart J* 2010;31:2915–57.
3. Warnes CA, Williams RG, Bashore TM et al. ACC/AHA 2008 guidelines for the management of adults with congenital heart disease. *J Am Coll Cardiol* 2008;52:e143–263.
4. Valente AM, Cook S, Festa P et al. Multimodality imaging guidelines for patients with repaired Tetralogy of Fallot. *J Am Soc Echocardiogr* 2014;27:111–41.

# Pericardial disease

## 15

- Echocardiography is requested for patients with known or suspected:
  - pericardial effusion (Table 15.1)
  - pericardial constriction
  - pericarditis.
- It may be used to guide percutaneous pericardial drainage.

**Table 15.1** Causes of pericardial effusions[1]

| Common | |
|---|---|
| Infection | Viral (Coxsackievirus, echovirus, HIV), TB, coxiella |
| Cancer | Angiosarcoma, metastases |
| Metabolic | Low albumin, hypothyroidism, renal failure |
| Reactive | Chest infections especially pneumococcal |
| Systemic inflammatory diseases | SLE, rheumatoid arthritis, Sjogren's syndrome, systemic sclerosis |
| Heart failure | |
| Idiopathic | |
| **Uncommon** | |
| Post radiation | |
| Dressler's syndrome | Autoimmune pericarditis after post cardiac surgery, myocardial infarction or trauma |
| Direct injury | Blunt or sharp chest injury, RF ablation |
| Drugs | Isoniazid, minoxidil, hydralazine, phenytoin |
| Aortic dissection | |

# Pericardial effusion

## 1 Pericardial or pleural?

- The differentiation is usually obvious (Table 15.2 and Figure 15.1). The key is where the effusion ends in relation to the descending thoracic aorta.

- The differentiation may be hard:
  - after cardiac surgery when localised posterior effusions may occur and extend a little over the left atrium
  - when there is extensive shielding behind the posterior aorta.
- Both pleural and pericardial effusions may coexist.

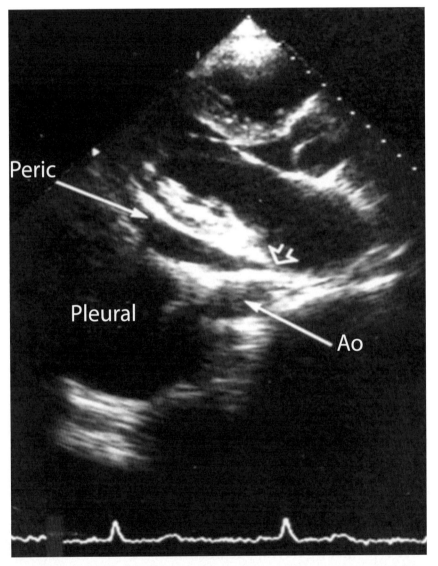

**Figure 15.1 Pericardial vs pleural fluid.** A pericardial effusion ends anterior to the descending thoracic aorta; a pleural effusion ends posterior to the aorta. A pleural effusion may extend over the left atrium; a pericardial effusion never does to any significant degree.

**Table 15.2** Differential diagnosis of pericardial and pleural effusions

| Pericardial | Pleural |
|---|---|
| Ends anterior to the descending aorta | Ends posterior to the descending aorta |
| Almost never overlaps left atrium | May overlap left atrium |
| Fluid between heart and diaphragm on subcostal view | No fluid between heart and diaphragm on subcostal view |
| Tamponade may be present | No signs of tamponade |
| Rarely >40 mm in depth | May often be >40mm |
| If large, swinging of the heart | Heart fixed |

## 2 Size and distribution

- Pericardial fluid is always present so a trivial effusion is usually normal especially around the right atrium.
- Size (Table 15.3) is less important than signs of tamponade (Table 15.4).
- Small effusions may cause tamponade if acute (e.g. after instrumentation of the heart) or if there is LV hypertrophy.

**Table 15.3** Grading of pericardial effusion size

| | |
|---|---|
| Trivial | Seen only in systole or localised around the RA |
| Small | <10 mm at end-diastole |
| Moderate | 10–20 mm at end diastole |
| Large | >20 mm at end diastole |

- Is the effusion generalised or localised, e.g. posterior, apical or anterior?
- Is there enough fluid in the subcostal view for safe pericardiocentesis (usually >20 mm but at least 10 mm)?
- What is the consistency of the fluid?
  - Echolucent
  - Localised strands which are common if the protein content is high and common in tuberculosis
  - Echodense. Haematomas occur after cardiac surgery, chest trauma and dissection
- Are there reasons why drainage with a needle might not be feasible?
  - Too small
  - Loculated
  - Echodense

## 3 Is tamponade present?

- Ultimately this is a clinical diagnosis but it is aided by the echocardiogram (Table 15.4).
- In ventilated patients the signs may be modified by mechanical ventilation. The decision to drain an effusion may be based on:
  - haemodynamic deterioration without other obvious cause, and
  - the presence of sufficient fluid on the echocardiogram to drain safely.

Table 15.4 Echocardiographic evidence of tamponade

| |
|---|
| Dilated IVC ( >20 mm ) with inspiratory collapse of <50% (Figure 15.2) |
| Fall in aortic or early diastolic mitral velocity during inspiration >25%[2] (Figure 15.3) |
| Increase in transtricuspid velocities on inspiration >40% |
| Prolonged and widespread diastolic right ventricular collapse (ideally recorded on M-mode to improve timing) |
| Shift of the ventricular septum to the left during inspiration |

NB Collapse of the right atrium and right ventricular outflow tract occur before RV collapse and are non-specific signs

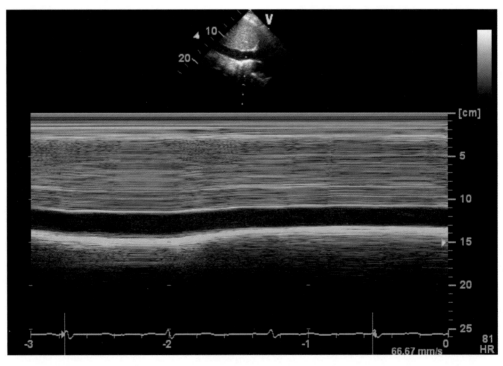

Figure 15.2 Engorged inferior vena cava. There is little change in diameter throughout the respiratory cycle or after a sniff.

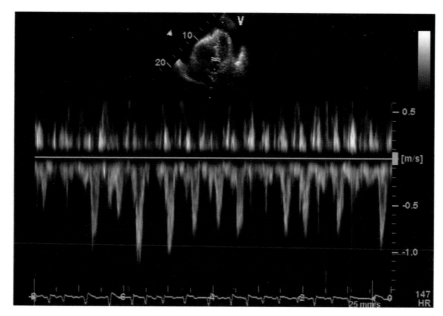

**Figure 15.3 Increased paradox.** This signal was recorded in a patient with tamponade. The subaortic peak velocity falls by >25% during inspiration.

- After cardiac surgery there may be tamponade as a result of haematoma compressing the atria. This may require TOE for diagnosis.
- If there is tamponade despite a small effusion (especially if chronic (>3 months), consider effusive-constrictive pericarditis. This requires investigation as for pericardial constriction.

## 4 Differential diagnoses

- The main differentials of pericardial fluid are:
  - pleural fluid
  - fat which most commonly occurs anteriorly or between the RV and diaphragm. It contains the appearance of fascial planes although there may also be echolucent fluid
  - a pericardial cyst may be large and resemble a localised effusion.
- Increased left-sided respiratory variation may also be caused by
  - asthma
  - right heart failure
  - underfilling.

## 5 LV function

- Is left ventricular function poor?
  - Pericardial effusion can complicate myocarditis.
  - Total pericardiocentesis may cause circulatory collapse.
  - Wall motion abnormalities may complicate tamponade even with normal coronary anatomy.

# Pericardial constriction

- This needs to be considered in patients with:
  - clinical evidence of heart failure but normal LV ejection fraction
  - any of the possible cause of pericardial constriction (Table 15.5).
- The key to the physiology is that the ventricles are normal but surrounded by a rigid 'box' causing:
  - increased ventricular interdependence (i.e. as the RV gets bigger on inspiration, the LV must get smaller)
  - on inspiration the fall in intrathoracic pressure is not transmitted inside the pericardium so pulmonary venous flow and therefore left-sided velocities drop.

Table 15.5 Causes of pericardial constriction

| |
|---|
| Tuberculosis |
| Radiation |
| Post viral |
| Rheumatoid arthritis |
| Idiopathic |
| After cardiac surgery (rare) |

## 1 Visual assessment

- **Septal bounce** (Figure 15.4). This may be the first clue that there is constrictive pericarditis. It is caused by an early diastolic pressure rise in the RV.[3]
- **Pericardial thickening.** This is not reliably detected or excluded on transthoracic echocardiography but extensive thickening may still alert the echocardiographer to the diagnosis. Thickness is better measured on CT.
- **LA size.** There is mild or moderate biatrial enlargement in pericardial constriction.
- **IVC.** This will be dilated with reduced contraction on inspiration.

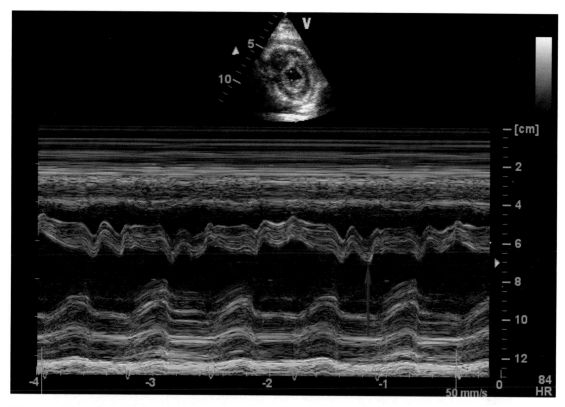

**Figure 15.4 Septal bounce.** This is an M-mode recording showing inward motion of the septum in systole but also diastole (the bounce (arrowed)).

And here's an electronic link to a loop on the website or use
http://goo.gl/lw5YNB

And here's an electronic link to a loop on the website or use
http://goo.gl/Qo7Jlz

## 2 Doppler

- **LV filling pattern**. This is characteristically restrictive (E:A ratio >2 and E deceleration time <150 ms) (Figure 15.5a).
- **Respiratory variability (spontaneous respiration).** Record the transmitral E wave or the peak transaortic velocities. Subtract the lowest (inspiratory) from

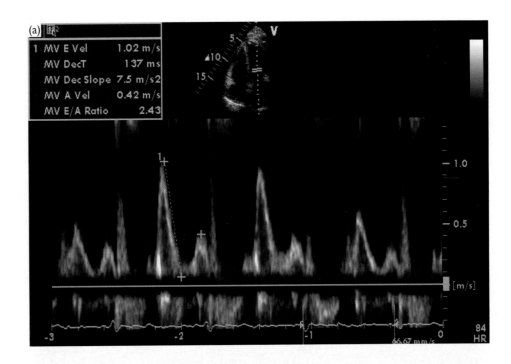

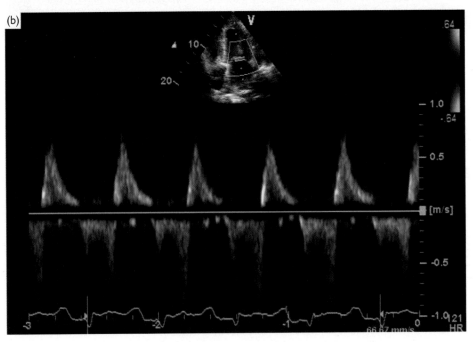

**Figure 15.5 Differentiating pericardial constriction and constrictive cardiomyopathy.** Image (a) was recorded in a patient with pericardial constriction. The transmitral E deceleration time was <140 ms and the peak E velocity fell by around 50% on inspiration. Image (b) was recorded in a patient with amyloid secondary to multiple myeloma between the second and fourth cycles shown. The E wave varies little throughout the respiratory cycle.

the highest (expiratory) and express as a percentage of the highest velocity. This is characteristically increased by >25% (Figure 15.5a).

- **Tissue Doppler.** LV function is normal so normal systolic velocities and normal or raised E′velocities are characteristic. The peak E′ velocity may be higher at the septal than the lateral annulus (which becomes tethered to the pericardium).
- **Estimated PA pressure.** This is moderately increased (usually <50 mmHg).
- **Hepatic vein flow.** Flow reversal is maximal on the first beat after expiration.
- **Pulmonary vein flow.** The systolic to diastolic (S:D) velocity ratio is >0.65 on inspiration and D velocity falls by >40% on inspiration.

## 3 Pericardial constriction or restrictive cardiomyopathy?

- Many of the causes of pericardial constriction also affect the myocardium so that these may coexist and it is necessary to determine which is dominant (Table 15.6).
- The key is that the ventricles are normal in constrictive pericarditis but abnormal in restrictive cardiomyopathy.
  - An E′ at the lateral or septal annulus of ≥8 cm/s differentiates constrictive pericarditis from restrictive cardiomyopathy.[4]
  - A low systolic velocity on TDI suggests restrictive cardiomyopathy, but may not be reliable.[4]
  - Respiratory variability is usually <10% in restrictive cardiomyopathy[2,5] (Figure 15.5b).
  - The LV may be hypertrophied and systolic function low normal in restrictive cardiomyopathy.

Table 15.6 Differentiating pericardial constriction and restrictive cardiomyopathy

| | Constriction | Restrictive myopathy |
|---|---|---|
| **Common to both** | | |
| Normal LV size and systolic function | | |
| Restrictive transmitral physiology (E:A >2 and E dec <150 ms) (Figure 15.5) | | |
| Dilated unreactive IVC (Figure 15.2) | | |
| **Points differentiating constriction and restrictive cardiomyopathy** | | |
| Fall in transmitral E velocity or aortic velocity on inspiration (Figure 15.5) | >25% | <10% |
| Tissue Doppler E′ | ≥8 cm/s | <7 |

(*continued*)

Table 15.6 Differentiating pericardial constriction and restrictive cardiomyopathy (*continued*)

|  | Constriction | Restrictive myopathy |
|---|---|---|
| LA and RA dilatation | Mild or moderate | Severe |
| Septal bounce (Figure 15.4) | Present | Absent |
| Hepatic flow reversal maximal | Expiration | Inspiration |
| PA systolic pressure | <50 mmHg | May be >50 mmHg |

## 4 Other techniques[6]

- CMR or CT is needed if a definitive diagnosis cannot be made on echocardiography.
- CT:
  - Measures pericardial thickness and detects calcification and masses
  - Evaluates the rest of the chest for evidence of malignancy and other lung pathology
  - Determines proximity of left internal mammary artery graft to sternum if a thoracotomy is being planned
  - Assesses coronary arteries
  - For imaging of LV, RV and atria if echocardiography suboptimal
- CMR:
  - Less accurate than CT for pericardial thickness but can show pericardial inflammation
  - Imaging of LV and atria if echocardiography suboptimal
  - Better tissue characterisation than echo for pericardial masses and for contents of the effusion (blood vs fluid) if not obvious echocardiographically
- Cardiac catheterisation:
  - If surgery is being planned, cardiac catheterisation allows contrast coronary angiography.
  - Restrictive physiology is confirmed by equalisation of diastolic pressures in all four chambers in constriction with concordance throughout the respiratory cycle and also concordance of the area under the pressure wave.

# Pericarditis

- Pericarditis is a clinical diagnosis based mainly on the characteristics of the pain, concave ST elevation in multiple arterial territories on the 12-lead ECG and the presence of a friction rub on auscultation.

- The role of echocardiography is to:
  - exclude myocarditis
  - detect pericardial fluid and tamponade
  - corroborate the diagnosis by showing a pericardial effusion and bright inflamed pericardium (but present in few cases)
  - detect clues to the diagnosis, e.g. valve involvement in SLE
  - exclude a wall motion abnormality if there is doubt whether the ST segment changes could be caused by an acute coronary syndrome.

 **MISTAKES TO AVOID**

- Failing to image subcostally to check that there is a sufficient depth of pericardial effusion to allow safe pericardiocentesis
- Forgetting to check for a septal 'bounce', dilated IVC and short transmitral E deceleration time in a patient with clinical heart failure but normal LV size and ejection fraction
- Diagnosing epicardial fat as a pericardial effusion

**CHECKLIST FOR REPORTING PERICARDIAL DISEASE**

1. Pericardial effusion:
   a. Size and site
   b. Consistency
   c. Is there fluid in the subcostal approach?
2. LV size and function including septal 'bounce'
3. RV collapse
4. Transmitral filling pattern
5. Respiratory variability
6. Tissue Doppler at the septal and lateral mitral annulus
7. PA pressure
8. IVC size and response to inspiration
9. Atrial size

# References

1.  Imazio M, Adler Y. Management of pericardial effusion. *Eur Heart J* 2013;34:1186–97.
2.  Goldstein JA. Cardiac tamponade, constrictive pericarditis, and restrictive cardiomyopathy. *Curr Prob Cardiol* 2004;29(9):503–67.
3.  Coylewright , Welch TD, Nishimura RA. Mechanism of septal bounce in constrictive pericarditis: a simultaneous cardiac catheterisation and echocardiographic study. *Heart* 2013;99:1376.
4.  Rajagopalan N, Garcia MJ, Rodriguez L et al. Comparison of new Doppler echocardiographic methods to differentiate constrictive pericardial heart disease and restrictive cardiomyopathy. *Am J Cardiol* 2001;87(1):86–94.
5.  Maisch B, Seferovic PM, Ristic AD et al. Guidelines on the diagnosis and management of pericardial diseases executive summary; The Task Force on the Diagnosis and Management of Pericardial Diseases of the European Society of Cardiology. *Eur Heart J* 2004;25(7):587–610.
6.  Klein AL, Abbara S, Agler DA et al. American Society of Echocardiography clinical recommendations for multimodality cardiovascular imaging of patients with pericardial disease. *J Am Soc Echocardiogr* 2013;26:965–1012.

# Masses

# 16

- Secondary tumours are at least 20 times more common than primary tumours.[1, 2]
- The most common benign primary tumours are atrial myxoma (70%), papillary fibroelastoma (10%), fibroma and, mainly in infants and children, rhabdomyoma.[1, 2]
- The most common primary malignancies are the sarcomas especially angiosarcomas which usually arise in the RA. Lymphomas are less common.

## 1 Describe the basic characteristics of the mass

The basic characteristics of a mass are listed in Table 16.1. The site of attachment and shape may be more easily appreciated using 3D.

Table 16.1 Characteristics of the mass

| Site and attachment |
| --- |
| Size, shape |
| Density (low intensity, dense, mixed) |
| Mobility (fixed, mobile, free) |
| Evidence of invasiveness |

## 2 A mass attached to a valve

- This can be rounded or thin (Table 16.2).
- It is not possible to differentiate reliably a vegetation from a myxomatous mitral valve with ruptured chords. The echocardiogram has to be interpreted within the clinical context.
- Echogenicity related to a valve annulus:
  - mitral annular calcification: occasionally large and mistaken for an abnormal mass
  - fat in the tricuspid annulus: this is normal.

Table 16.2 Masses attached to valves

| Native valves | |
|---|---|
| **Rounded** | |
| Vegetation | *Infective:* Occur on any valve, usually move independently of the valve and are associated with valve destruction |
| | *Libman-Sacks in SLE or isolated antiphospholipid syndrome:* Usually broad-based <10 mm in diam attached to aortic or mitral valves and associated with generalised valve thickening. May be calcified when chronic |
| | *Malignant:* Indistinguishable from infective vegetations but less likely to be associated with valve destruction |
| | *Other:* Rheumatoid arthritis |
| Fibroelastoma | Small (usually <10mm) with a short stalk, rounded with fronds often with mixed echogenicity. Attached to the aortic more than the mitral valve, and less commonly pulmonary or tricuspid (or mitral or tricuspid chordae) (Figure 16.1) |
| Myxomatous tissue | Usually generalised mild 'fleshiness' associated with prolapse but may be florid in Barlow's syndrome. Mainly affect the mitral valve, less commonly the tricuspid valve |
| Calcific deposit | The edges of atherosclerotic degeneration may be 'furry' or occasionally pedunculated |
| **Thin** | |
| Single ruptured chord | This produces a whip-like appearance most often seen in the LA and moving between LA and LV |
| Fibrin strand | Also called Lambl's excrescences. These are attached to the closure line of the aortic valve |
| **Replacement valves** | |
| **Solid** | |
| Thrombus | This is more common in mechanical valves and requires TOE for full delineation |
| Vegetation | These may be attached to the cusps of a biological valve or the sewing ring of any design |
| Other | In old valves, disruption of the fabric covering the sewing ring or endothelial tags can rarely cause non-infected masses attached to the sewing ring |
| **Thin** | |
| Stitch | These may be obvious around the sewing ring on TOE, occasionally on TTE |
| Fibrin strand | These are seen mainly in mechanical valves in either main position and consist of 10–20 mm mobile strands attached to the leaflets |

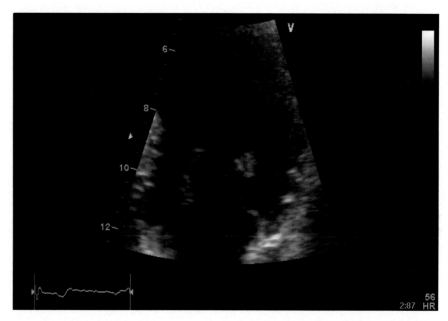

**Figure 16.1 Fibroelastoma.** An apical 4-chamber view showing a small pedunculated mass of mixed echogenicity attached to the posterior leaflet of the mitral valve.

And here's an electronic link to a loop on the website or use
http://goo.gl/X6G9Lf

## 3 Left or right atrial mass

- Many apparent masses are normal (Table 16.3). Pathological masses are listed in Table 16.4.
- For an RA mass:
  - An associated pericardial effusion suggests an angiosarcoma (Figure 16.2).
  - Check the IVC for tumour extension from a primary in the kidneys, liver, uterus or ovaries.
  - Thrombus from a deep vein thrombosis may also appear in the IVC. Typically, a tumour will cause IVC dilatation (Figure 16.3) while a thrombus will not.
- For an LA mass:
  - If immobile and attached to the wall, check the pulmonary veins and look for a tumour mass outside the heart.
  - Thrombus is unlikely without a substrate (dilated left atrium, mitral stenosis, atrial fibrillation).

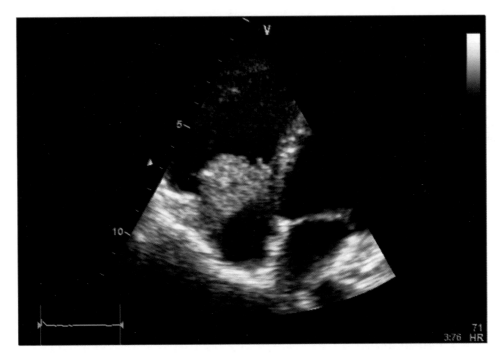

**Figure 16.2 Angiosarcoma.** An off-axis 4-chamber view showing a mass attached to the free wall of the right atrium. This is the most common malignant cardiac tumour and may often be associated with a pericardial effusion.

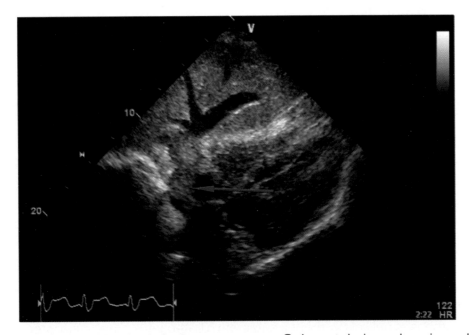

**Figure 16.3 Tumour in the inferior vena cava.** Subcostal view showing a large tumour mass stretching the inferior vena cava and entering the right atrium.

And here's an electronic link to a loop on the website or use
http://goo.gl/5YB8z6

And here's an electronic link to a loop on the website or use
http://goo.gl/lyfK0e

Table 16.3 Non-pathological atrial 'masses'

| | |
|---|---|
| Eustachian valve | Attached at the opening of the IVC, this can be fixed or mobile, thin or thick and up to 20 mm in length |
| Chiari membrane or net | Attached between the Eustachian valve and the atrial septum; thin and may move gently |
| Atrial septal aneurysm | The apex may initially be seen as an apparent mass in the LA in parasternal long-axis views although the diagnosis is obvious in other views |
| Atrial septal fat | This is deposited in a dumb-bell shape at either end of the septum and sparing the centre |
| Pacemaker electrode | Sections of the electrode will lie outside the plane of the ultrasound so this requires multiple views |
| Long central line | Usually the 'railway track' appearance of the cannula is obvious |

Table 16.4 Pathological atrial masses

| | |
|---|---|
| Intracavitary | *Fixed* band across LA in cor triatriatum |
| | *Mobile* mass in RA: thrombus or tumour entering via IVC or thrombus wedged in PFO |
| | *Free-floating* ball thrombus in the LA (associated AF and mitral stenosis) |
| Septum | *Myxoma:* Attached at the centre on the left much more commonly than right. Mixed echogenicity. When large, may prolapse through the MV in diastole or prevent full closure in systole |
| | *Thrombus:* A vein cast may become embedded in a PFO and may have elements in RA and LA cavities |
| Left atrial appendage (LAA) | 95% of LA thrombus starts here and may be seen in a 2-chamber apical view |

*(continued)* *(continued)*

Table 16.4 Pathological atrial masses (*continued*)

| Wall | *Thrombus:* Commonly around the LAA or at the most basal part of the LA between the right and left veins or of the RA between the IVC and SVC in a 4-chamber view |
|------|------|
|  | *Tumour:* A sessile immobile mass attached to the free wall of the RA is often an angiosarcoma (Figure 16.2) |

## 4 Left and right ventricular mass

See Table 16.5.

- An associated pericardial effusion suggests that the mass is malignant.
- LV thrombus is rare without an underlying structural abnormality (e.g. dilated LV, hypertrabeculation) but may occur in a normal LV with thrombophilia (e.g. primary biliary cirrhosis, Behçet's syndrome).
- RV thrombus may complicate deep-vein thrombosis or occur as a complication of an RV myopathy.

Table 16.5 Causes of LV or RV masses

| Intracavitary | |
|------|------|
| Thrombus | Characteristics on Table 16.6, page 185 |
| Endomyocardial fibrosis | Causes thrombus at the apex of RV and LV which may extend to the base of the heart and involve the AV valves |
| Hypertrabeculation | Occur predominantly in noncompaction (Figure 4.3, page 40) |
| Benign tumours | Fibroelastomas and myxoma may occasionally occur in the LV or RV |
| **Solely or predominantly intramyocardial** | |
| Metastasis | Occur anywhere in the LV or RV wall and may then extend inwards or outwards. Most commonly breast, lung, gastric and colonic. Also characteristic with rare tumours: melanoma, germ cell, thymoma |
| Primary malignancy | Lymphomas or sarcomas extend outwards and may be associated with a pericardial effusion |
| Fibroma | Usually in septum or LV free wall. May be up to 100 mm in diameter. Characteristic central calcification (Figure 16.4) |
| Rhabdomyoma | Multiple bright intramural masses often extending into the cavity. Usually resolve in childhood |
| Systemic disease | Myocardial nodules can occur in sarcoid, tuberculosis or rheumatoid arthritis |
| Hydatid disease | Cystic, semisolid or solid. Single or multiple. Also seen in the pericardium |

- Characteristics of thrombus are given in Table 16.6. If uncertain, use different views and consider transpulmonary contrast.
- Could the mass be normal (Table 16.7)?

**Table 16.6** Features of thrombus

| |
|---|
| Underlying wall motion abnormality |
| Cleavage plane between thrombus and LV wall |
| Higher density than myocardium |
| Present in more than one view |
| Causes a void on colour mapping or contrast echocardiography |

**Table 16.7** Normal LV or RV 'masses'

| | |
|---|---|
| Trabeculation | Trabeculation is a feature of the RV and minor trabeculation is also common in the LV. It increases with athletic training, especially in black athletes |
| Prominent moderator band | Normal feature of the RV |
| LV false tendon | Runs parallel with the septal endocardium |
| Prominent papillary muscle | An occasional cause of confusion resolved by following back the apparent mass to show continuity with LV wall and chordae |
| Aberrant papillary muscle | Ectopic extra papillary tissue is sometimes seen, e.g. in the LV outflow tract |
| Near-field effects at apex | Not seen in every view. Resolves with changes in focus and gain. Occasionally need contrast to resolve |

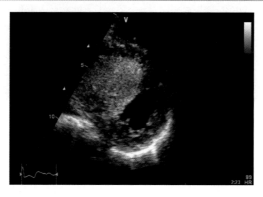

**Figure 16.4 Fibroma.** Parasternal short-axis view showing a large intramyocardial mass which is distinct from the surrounding myocardium.

 And here's an electronic link to a loop on the website or use
http://goo.gl/iW0932

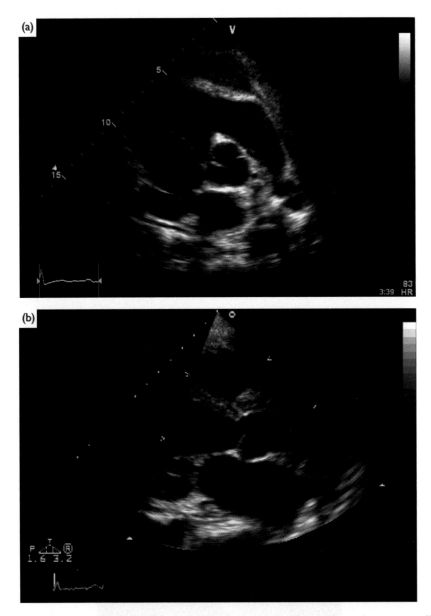

Figure 16.5   Lymphoma. A parasternal short-axis view showing a mediastinal mass (a) that extends down the anterior aorta in a long-axis view (b).

And here's an electronic link to a loop on the website or use
http://goo.gl/vt0xV4

## 5 Extrinsic masses

See Table 16.8.

Table 16.8 Masses outside the heart

| Abnormal findings | |
| --- | --- |
| Mediastinal tumour | Lymphoma (Figure 16.5) |
| Lymph node | Often seen adjacent to the pulmonary artery |
| Haematoma | |
| Pericardial cyst | |
| Pericardial hydatid | May be single or multiloculated or solid |
| Pseudoaneurysm | Not usually a diagnostic problem with an associated myocardial infarct |
| Subdiaphragmatic masses | Cysts in the liver or kidney |
| Normal findings confused with masses | |
| Descending thoracic aorta | |
| Hiatus hernia | This is of mixed echogenicity |
| Back bone | This may be especially prominent in a patient with a pectus excavatum |
| Pericardial fat | Seen most commonly anteriorly in a parasternal long-axis view and between the diaphragm and RV subcostally |

## 6 Masses in the great vessels

See Table 16.9.

Table 16.9 Masses in the great arteries

| Pulmonary artery | |
| --- | --- |
| Thrombus | Associated with deep-vein thrombosis and pulmonary embolism (Table 17.2, page 192) |
| Sarcoma | Rare |
| Myxoma | Very rare |
| Aortic | |
| Dissection | The serpiginous movement of a flap in a dilated aorta is usually obvious, but a localised dissection after instrumentation may produce a small focal thickening |

(*continued*)

Table 16.9 Masses in the great arteries (*continued*)

| Pulmonary artery | |
|---|---|
| Pedunculated atheroma | Most commonly seen on TOE |
| Fungal aortitis | Rare complication of cardiac surgery but classical appearance of large vegetation attached to the aortic wall at the site of the aortotomy |

## 7 Haemodynamic effect

Assess the presence and degree of valve regurgitation or obstruction to inflow depending on the site of the mass.

## 8 Other features

Certain features may aid the diagnosis of the mass:
● Presence of a pericardial effusion suggesting malignancy
● Substrate for thrombus formation:
  ● AF
  ● enlarged LA
  ● mitral stenosis
  ● dilated hypokinetic LV
● Medical history e.g. cancer, pulmonary embolism, evidence of infective endocarditis

## 9 Other techniques

If characterisation is difficult, consider other techniques (Table 16.10).

Table 16.10 Other techniques for characterising cardiac masses

| Technique | Value |
|---|---|
| Contrast echo<br>● confirming presence and site<br>● demonstrating vascularity | |
| TOE | Improved characterisation of all atrial masses |
| CMR<br>● improved tissue characterisation<br>● differentiates thrombus from myxoma<br>● can confirm presence of cardiac lipomas<br>● perfusion (vascularity of masses) | |

| Technique | Value |
|-----------|-------|
| PET | Demonstrating metabolic activity in malignancy and involvement of other organs |
| CT | Mediastinal extent and involvement of other organs. Demonstrates local invasion |

 ## MISTAKES TO AVOID

- Overdiagnosing normal variants as abnormal
- Failing to check the IVC if there is a right atrial mass
- Ignoring the clinical background when suggesting the nature of a mass, e.g. the presence of atrial fibrillation especially with atrial or LV dilatation makes thrombus more likely than tumour

### CHECKLIST FOR REPORTING A MASS

1. Location and site of attachment
2. Size and density
3. Mobility
4. Involvement of adjacent veins
5. Evidence of invasion
6. Haemodynamic effect
7. Is there a pericardial effusion?
8. Is there a substrate for thrombus?

## References

1. Lam KY, Dickens P, Chan AC. Tumors of the heart: a 20-year experience with a review of 12485 consecutive autopsies. *Arch Pathol Lab Med* 1993;117:1027–31.
2. Butany J, Nair V, Naseemuddin A, Nair GM, Catton C, Yau T. Cardiac tumours: diagnosis and management. *Lancet Oncol* 2005;6:219–28.
3. Auger D, Pressacco J, Marcotte F, Tremblay A, Dore A, Ducharme A. Cardiac masses: an integrative approach using echocardiography and other imaging modalities. *Heart* 2011;97:1101–9.

# Echocardiography in acute and critical care medicine

## 17

Standard echocardiography is vital in many acute presentations. However, the patient may be critically ill and require an abbreviated scan to help make potentially life-saving clinical decisions.

- A number of basic focused ultrasound protocols have been developed for the emergency department, critical care units or the periarrest situation, e.g. FEEL, FATE, FICE, FUSE, FOCUS, ELS, USLS, FAST, CFEU, ACC/AHA. Most of these include the heart alone, while others also include the lungs or abdomen.
- Echocardiography is increasingly used for the assessment of acutely ill patients as effectively an extension of the clinical examination. Protocols are still being developed[1, 2] but often have these features:
  - Include colour as well as imaging to detect significant valve disease
  - Use standard basic views, e.g. parasternal long- and short-axis, apical 4-and 5-chamber, subcostal
  - Look systematically at all key cardiac structures:
    - LV size and function
    - RV size and function
    - IVC
    - valves
    - presence of pericardial fluid

## 1 Indications for immediate ultrasound scanning

The following checklists indicate features identifiable using a limited study but also those requiring a more detailed standard study (marked with *).

- Cardiac arrest (Table 17.1). The aim is to detect reversible causes (e.g. tamponade, pulmonary embolism, severe hypovolemia) and also pathology suggesting that prolonged resuscitation is likely to be futile (e.g. cardiac rupture)
- Clinically likely pulmonary embolism and patient still hypotensive 1 hour after heparin. The treatment might be thrombolysis if the RV is dilated and the PA systolic pressure high (Table 17.2)
- Unexplained severe hypotension (Table 17.3)
- Unexplained pulmonary oedema (Table 17.4)
- Haemodynamically unstable after myocardial infarction (Table 17.1)
- Chest pain where aortic dissection or pulmonary embolism is possible (Table 17.2)

- Trauma in the following circumstances (Table 17.5):
  - unexplained clinical deterioration
  - serious blunt or penetrating chest trauma
  - deceleration or crush injuries
  - widening of the mediastinum or suspected aortic injury (also consider TOE or CT)
- Acute exacerbation of COPD. While not usually a critical emergency, 20% may have LV failure[3] so that early echocardiography may lead to an important change in management

**Table 17.1** Checklist for echocardiography in cardiac arrest

| |
|---|
| Critical LV dysfunction |
| Acute complications of infarction:<br>• Papillary muscle rupture<br>• Ventricular septal rupture*<br>• Free wall rupture* |
| LV hypertrophy suggesting HCM |
| Right ventricular dilatation (see Table 17.2) |
| Pericardial tamponade |
| Critical valve disease especially aortic stenosis |
| Obstructed prosthetic valve* |
| Aortic dissection rupturing into pleural space or abdominal cavity* |
| Gross hypovolemia - see also Table 17.3 |

*Likely to require a standard echocardiogram

**Table 17.2** Echocardiographic signs of pulmonary embolism with haemodynamic instability[4–6]

| |
|---|
| RV dilatation and free wall hypokinesis often with preserved contraction at the apex (McConnell's sign) |
| D-shaped LV in parasternal short-axis view |
| TR $V_{max}$ usually <4.0 m/s* |
| Short time to peak PA velocity <90 ms* |
| IVC dilated and unreactive |
| Occasionally thrombus in the pulmonary artery or right heart* |

*Requires a standard echocardiogram

Table 17.3 Checklist in hypotension

| Signs of underfilling |
|---|
| IVC <10 mm in diameter collapsing completely on inspiration |
| Small and active RV and LV ('kissing papillary muscles') |
| Low E and A wave on transmitral pulsed Doppler* |
| Respiratory variability in $VTI_{subaortic}$ >20% (in the absence of other pathology particularly pericardial effusion, RV dilatation or asthma)* |
| **Cardiogenic causes** |
| LV global or regional systolic dysfunction* |
| Dynamic LV outflow tract obstruction |
| RV dysfunction (see also Table 17.2) |
| Pericardial tamponade |
| Severe valve lesions |
| IVC diameter >20 mm and engorged |
| **Sepsis[7]** |
| LV either normal size or dilated with global hypokinesis or normal size and hyperdynamic (depending on fluid-loading and use of inotropes) |
| RV mildly dilated and hypokinetic (in the presence of Adult Respiratory Distress Syndrome) |

* Likely to require a standard echocardiogram

Table 17.4 Unexplained pulmonary oedema

| |
|---|
| Impaired LV function |
| Complications of a myocardial infarction: <br> • Papillary muscle rupture <br> • Ventricular septal rupture* <br> • Contained free wall rupture |
| Severe native valve disease |
| Thrombosed replacement mechanical heart valve* (may need TOE) |

* Likely to require a standard echocardiogram

Table 17.5 Checklist for echocardiography after blunt or penetrating trauma

| Blunt |
|---|
| Pericardial effusion |
| Contusion: <br> • RV dilatation and hypokinesis <br> • Localised LV thickening and wall motion abnormality especially anteroapically |

193

(*continued*)

Table 17.5 Checklist for echocardiography after blunt or penetrating trauma (*continued*)

| Blunt |
| --- |
| Ventricular septal rupture |
| Regional wall motion abnormality (from coronary artery dissection) |
| Valve rupture causing acute mitral or tricuspid regurgitation, occasionally aortic regurgitation |
| Aortic dilatation and dissection flap or intramural haematoma (TOE) |
| Aortic transection (TOE) |
| **Penetrating** |
| RV wall hypokinesis |
| Ventricular septal defect |
| Pericardial effusion or haematoma (which may be localised) |
| Pleural fluid |
| Mitral regurgitation from valve laceration or damage to papillary muscle or chordae |
| Aortic regurgitation from laceration of aortic valve |
| Hyperdynamic LV (from off-loading) |

## 2 Further indications for echocardiography on critical care units

The haemodynamic assessment of the heart may be affected by mechanical ventilation (Table 17.6).

- The diagnosis of tamponade is more clinically based than in a spontaneously breathing patient. In the presence of a pericardial effusion, a fall in blood pressure or cardiac output and/or the development of acute renal failure with no other reasonable cause should prompt consideration of drainage.
- Stopping ventilation transiently may clarify the haemodynamic state if high airway pressures or high positive end expiratory pressure (PEEP) settings are used.

The following situations require standard echocardiography, often with TOE.

- Hypotension after cardiac surgery (Table 17.7)
- Estimation of filling pressures, low in Table 17.3 and high in Table 17.8
- Assessment of likely cardiac output response to increased filling:
  - The response of the IVC and the $VTI_{subaortic}$ variation to standard leg raising aids the decision
  - In one study[8] fluid responsiveness was likely if the IVC had an 18% variation during controlled ventilation with specific ventilator settings calculated as:
    - 100 (IVC $Diam_{max}$ − IVC $Diam_{min}$)/ IVC $Diam_{min}$

- No universal echocardiographic threshold exists and the decision is made including numerous clinical factors
- Other common indications for echocardiography are given in Table 17.9
- Assessment for patients on ECMO (Appendix 2, Tables A2.1–A2.3), Impella device (Appendix 2, Table A2.4) and intra-aortic balloon pumps (Appendix 2, Table A2.5)

**Table 17.6** Effects of mechanical ventilation[9]

| |
|---|
| The timing of paradox is reversed in comparison to spontaneous ventilation with the left-sided fall of cardiac output occurring during the expiratory phase and a decrease in venous return on the right side during inspiration |
| Respiratory variation may be greater than normal depending on the inspiratory pressure, but if >25%:<br>• check ventilation settings<br>• exclude a pericardial effusion<br>• check LV and RV size and function<br>• check for hypovolaemia |
| High positive end-expiratory pressure (PEEP) around 10 mmHg reduces venous return and afterload. Its effect on LV systolic and diastolic function varies depending on whether there is pre-existing LV dysfunction but includes:<br>• reduced stroke volume<br>• reduced E′<br>• lengthening of E deceleration time |
| High-frequency oscillation ventilation causes an engorged IVC in all hearts |

**Table 17.7** Additional checklist for echocardiography in hypotension after cardiac surgery

| |
|---|
| All variables in Table 17.3 |
| HCM-like physiology after aortic valve replacement for aortic stenosis with small LV cavity, systolic anterior mitral valve motion and LV outflow acceleration |
| Systolic anterior mitral motion after mitral valve repair |
| Replacement valve regurgitation/ paraprosthetic leak or obstruction (TOE) |
| Native valve function |
| Localised haematoma over atria (TOE) or small effusion elsewhere causing acute tamponade |
| RV stunning post bypass and or ischaemia (air in right coronary artery) |

**Table 17.8** Signs of high filling pressures

| High RA pressure |
|---|
| IVC >20 mm in diameter and unresponsive (except with ventilation using high-frequency oscillation) or unreactive SVC on TOE |
| Dilated right atrium |
| Atrial septum bulges to the left (in the absence of severe tricuspid regurgitation) |
| **High LA pressure** |
| E/E' ratio >15 |
| E deceleration time <150 ms |
| Atrial septum bulges to the right (in the absence of mitral regurgitation) |
| Dilated left atrium if filling pressure chronically high |

**Table 17.9** Other common indications for echocardiography on critical care units

| Indication | Checklist* |
|---|---|
| Inability to wean from ventilator | LV and RV function, diastolic dysfunction, severe valve disease |
| | Pericardial effusion |
| Unexplained hypoxaemia | Evidence of pulmonary embolism (Table 17.2) |
| | Shunt (may require bubble study) (pages 145–146) |
| ARDS not responding to first-line measures | RV size and function |
| | PA pressures |
| Pre- and peri-administration of nitric oxide | RV function and PA pressures |
| Pre- and post-inotrope | LV and RV function |
| Possible endocarditis | Chapter 11 |
| Embolic event | Table 18.3 |

*A full study looking for abnormalities in all parts of the heart is needed

# References

1. Spencer KT, Kimura BJ, Korcarz CE et al. Focused cardiac ultrasound: recommendations from the American Society of Echocardiography. *J Am Soc Echocardiogr* 2013;26:567–81.
2. Victor K, Rajani R, Bruemmer-Smith S, Kabir S, Chambers J. A training programme in screening echocardiography. *Clin Teach* 2013;10(3):176–80. doi:10.1111/tct.12019.
3. Rutten FH, Cramer M-JM, Grobbee DE et al. Unrecognised heart failure in elderly patients with stable chronic obstructive pulmonary disease. *Eur Heart J* 2005;26:1887–94.
4. Kasper W, Geibel A, Tiede N et al. Distinguishing between acute and subacute massive pulmonary embolism by conventional and Doppler echocardiography. *Br Heart J* 1993;70:352–6.
5. Kjaergaard J, Schaadt BK, Lund JO, Hassager C. Quantitative measure of right ventricular dysfunction by echocardiography in the diagnosis of acute nonmassive pulmonary embolism. *J Am Soc Echocardiogr* 2006;19:1264–71.
6. McConnell MV, Solomon SD, Rayan ME, Come PC, Goldhaber SZ, Lee RT. Regional right ventricular dysfunction detected by echocardiography in acute pulmonary embolism. *Am J Cardiol* 1996;78:469–63.
7. Etchecopar-Chevreuil C, Francois B, Clavel M et al. Cardiac morphological and functional changes during early septic shock: a transesophageal echocardiographic study. *Int Care Med* 2008;34:250–6.
8. Barbier C, Loubieres Y, Schmit C et al. Respiratory changes in inferior vena cava diameter are helpful in predicting fluid responsiveness in ventilated septic patients. *Int Care Med* 2004;30:1740–6.
9. Chin JH, Lee EH, Choi DK, Hahm KD, Sim JY, Choi IC. Positive end-expiratory pressure aggravates left ventricular diastolic relaxation further in patients with pre-existing relaxation abnormalities. *Br J Anaesth* 2013;111(3):368–73. doi:10.1093/bja/aet061.

# General clinical requests

## 18

These tables give a guide on what to assess in various common indications for echocardiography not yet covered:

- Murmur (Table 18.1)
- Heart failure (Table 18.2)
- Stroke, TIA and peripheral embolism (Table 18.3)
- Cardiac arrhythmia (Table 18.4)
- Hypertension (Table 18.5)
- Cocaine (Table 18.6)
- HIV (Table 18.7)
- Neuromuscular diseases (Table 18.8)
- Inflammatory diseases (Table 18.9)
- Hypereosinophilia (Table 18.10)
- Drugs causing valvopathy (cabergoline, pergolide, benfluorex) (Table 18.11)
- Radiation (Table 18.12) mainly after treatment for non-Hodgkin's lymphoma or left-sided breast cancer more than 20 years ago
- Chagas disease (Table 18.13), which is beginning to be seen outside South America as a result of migration

**Table 18.1** Checklist in 'murmur'

| |
|---|
| Valve thickening or regurgitation |
| Subaortic septal bulge |
| ASD: clue is dilated active RV |
| VSD:<br>• parasternal long- and short-axis views with colour box on the membranous septum detect most<br>• colour box over the muscular septum in parasternal long and short and apical 4-chamber view<br>• apical septal defects may be missed (put CW probe over the site of the maximum murmur) |
| Coarctation (suprasternal view) |
| Continuous wave in pulmonary artery |
| PDA (parasternal short and suprasternal views) |

Table 18.2 Checklist in suspected 'heart failure'

| |
|---|
| LV cavity size and wall thickness and systolic and diastolic function |
| RV morphology, size and function |
| Indexed LA volume (as a sign of chronically high LV filling pressures) |
| IVC size and response to respiration |
| Valve appearance and function |

Table 18.3 Checklist in stroke, TIA or peripheral embolism[1]

| |
|---|
| LV global hypokinesis, aneurysm or large regional wall motion abnormality |
| Signs of hypertension (as the underlying cause of generalised vascular disease): LV hypertrophy, diastolic dysfunction, dilated LA, aortic sclerosis, aortic dilatation |
| Dilated LA |
| Evidence of aortic dissection: dilated aorta, dissection flap |
| Mitral valve disease: stenosis > regurgitation |
| ASD or patent foramen ovale (bubble study according to clinical indications usually in patients aged <50 years) |
| Masses: LA myxoma or thrombus, LV thrombus, valve vegetation or fibroelastoma |
| Atrial fibrillation (should already have been detected on the 12-lead ECG) |

Table 18.4a Checklist after ventricular tachycardia

| |
|---|
| LV size and systolic function |
| LV hypertrophy? |
| RV dysplasia (see pages 41–44) |
| Valve disease |

Table 18.4b Checklist in atrial fibrillation

| |
|---|
| Left and right atrial size |
| LV size and function |
| Mitral valve appearance and function |
| LA thrombus? |
| RV size and function |
| PA pressures |

Table 18.5 Checklist in hypertension

| LV hypertrophy (subaortic septal bulge may be an early sign) |
| --- |
| LV cavity size and systolic function |
| Systolic anterior motion of the anterior mitral leaflet (rare) |
| LV diastolic function |
| LA size |
| Aortic dimensions |
| Coarctation |
| Unfolding of the arch |
| Aortic valve thickening |

Table 18.6 Checklist in cocaine[2]

| **Acute** |
| --- |
| Wall motion abnormality (myocardial infarction) |
| Generalised LV hypokinesis (myocarditis) |
| Aortic dissection |
| **Long-term use** |
| Dilated LV |
| LV hypertrophy |
| Evidence of endocarditis |

Table 18.7 Checklist in HIV[3]

| Dilated left ventricle |
| --- |
| Pulmonary hypertension |
| Pericardial effusion |
| Evidence of endocarditis (increased susceptibility to infection) |
| Pericardial thickening (e.g. Kaposi sarcoma, non-Hodgkin's lymphoma) |

Table 18.8 Echocardiographic abnormalities in neuromuscular disorders[4, 5]

| Duchenne's muscular dystrophy | LV systolic dysfunction (starts inferoposteriorly) Pulmonary hypertension and RV dysfunction (secondary to respiratory failure) |
| --- | --- |
| Becker | LV dilatation (starts inferoposteriorly) |
| Fascioscapulohumeral | Usually no involvement |

(*continued*)

Table 18.8 Echocardiographic abnormalities in neuromuscular disorders (*continued*)

| Myotonic dystrophy | Cardiomyopathy uncommon (may be subclinical minor dysfunction on echo) |
|---|---|
| Emery–Dreifuss | Cardiomyopathy moderately common |
| Limb girdle dystrophy | Cardiomyopathy moderately common |
| Friedreich's ataxia | LV hypertrophy |
| **Mitochondrial myopathies** | |
| MELAS | Moderate risk of HCM |
| MERRF | Moderate risk of dilated cardiomyopathy or asymmetric septal hypertrophy |
| Kearns–Sayre | Low risk of dilated myopathy. May be mitral and tricuspid prolapse |

Table 18.9 Checklist in systemic inflammatory diseases[6, 7]

| Systemic lupus erythematosus (SLE) | LV dysfunction secondary to myocarditis |
|---|---|
| | Generalised valve thickening and vegetations (mitral and aortic most commonly affected) with regurgitation (stenosis very rare) |
| | Pulmonary hypertension |
| | Pericardial effusion (tamponade uncommon) |
| Primary antiphospholipid syndrome | Generalised valve thickening and vegetations (mitral and aortic most commonly affected) with regurgitation (stenosis very rare) |
| | Right-sided thrombus |
| | Pulmonary hypertension |
| | LV dysfunction (secondary to systemic hypertension or coronary disease) |
| Rheumatoid arthritis | Nodules typically at base of leaflets |
| | Valve thickening commonly focal and mild but may be diffuse |
| Ankylosing spondylitis | Aortic root dilatation with thickening and fibrosis of the base of the aortic cusps and anterior mitral leaflet |
| Wegener's | Aortic valve vegetations with regurgitation |
| | Pericarditis |
| | LV systolic dysfunction |
| | Aortic aneurysms |

| Churg–Strauss | Myocarditis common |
|---|---|
| | Pericardial effusion |
| Systemic sclerosis (scleroderma) | Myocardial fibrosis leading to diastolic > systolic LV failure |
| | Pulmonary hypertension and RV failure (secondary to lung fibrosis) |
| | Pericardial effusion (c40%) |
| | Aortic or mitral valve thickening (c10%) |
| Polymyositis/dermatomyositis | LV diastolic dysfunction (c40%) |
| | Pulmonary hypertension (interstitial lung disease) |
| Mixed connective tissue disease | Pulmonary hypertension |
| Sjogren syndrome | Cardiac involvement uncommon |
| | Pulmonary hypertension (secondary to lung involvement) |
| Behçet's disease | Myocarditis |
| | RA and RV thrombus |
| | Pulmonary artery aneurysms |
| Cogan's disease | Aortic dilatation and aortic regurgitation |
| Sarcoidosis | Dilated myopathy or regional scarring |
| | Localised nodules |
| Takayasu's arteritis | Aortic dilatation with secondary aortic regurgitation |
| | Pulmonary artery dilatation |
| | Pulmonary stenosis |
| | Fistulae between pulmonary artery and coronary or bronchial arteries or aorta |
| | Subclinical myocardial involvement |
| Giant cell arteritis | Thoracic aortic aneurysm |
| Polyarteritis nodosa | Dilated cardiomyopathy |
| Microscopic polyangiitis | Heart failure |
| | Pericarditis |
| Kawasaki | Myocardial infarction |
| | Myocarditis and pericarditis acutely |

**Table 18.10** Checklist in hypereosinophilia, Loeffler's endocarditis, endomyocardial fibrosis

| |
|---|
| Hyperdense endocardium |
| LV and RV apical thrombus (Figure 4.2, page 38) |
| Fibrous attachment of tricuspid and mitral valves |

**Table 18.11** Checklist in drug treatment with cabergoline, pergolide, benfluorex

| |
|---|
| May affect mitral, aortic or tricuspid valves |
| Thickening, restriction and regurgitation |
| First sign may be increased tenting height of the mitral valve |
| The thickening affects the whole the leaflet |
| Almost never seen with low dose cabergoline used in microprolactinoma |

**Table 18.12** Checklist in radiation[9]

| | |
|---|---|
| Valve disease | Thickening of the aortic and mitral valves |
| | Regurgitation more common than stenosis |
| | Incidence 6% 20 years after irradiation |
| LV dysfunction | Diffuse myocardial fibrosis |
| | Initially systolic dysfunction, later restrictive myopathy |
| Coronary disease | Regional wall motion abnormalities |
| Pericardial constriction | Incidence 4–20% depending on dose and concomitant use of chemotherapy |

**Table 18.13** Checklist in Chagas disease[10]

| |
|---|
| Regional wall motion abnormalities especially posteroinferior (20% asymptomatic but up to 30% with symptoms) |
| Apical aneurysm (8% in asymptomatic patients but up to 60% in those with breathlessness) |
| Generalised LV dilatation and hypokinesis in advanced disease |

# References

1. Pepi M, Evangelista A, Nihoyannopouls P et al. Recommendations for echocardiography use in the diagnosis and management of cardiac sources of embolism. *Eur J Echocardiogr* 2010;11:461–76.
2. Missouris CG, Swift PA, Singer DRJ. Cocaine use and acute left ventricular dysfunction. *Lancet* 2001;357:1586.

3. Lipshultz SE, Fisher SD, Miller TL, Sharma TS, Milton AN. The cardiovascular manifestations of HIV infection. *Dialog Cardiovasc Med* 2007;12:5–23.

4. Bouhouch R, Elhouari T, Oukerraj L et al. Management of cardiac involvement in neuromuscular diseases: review. *Open Cardiovas Med J* 2008;2:93–6.

5. Barrera-Ramirez CF, Barragán-Campos HM, Ilarraza H, Iturralde P, Ávila-Casado MC, Oseguerab J. Cardiac involvement in Kearns–Sayre Syndrome. *Rev Esp Cardiol* 2005;58:443–6.

6. Roldan CA. Valvular and coronary heart disease in systemic inflammatory diseases. *Heart* 2008;94:1089–101.

7. Ferri C, Giuggioli D, Sebastiani M et al. Heart involvement and systemic sclerosis. *Lupus* 2005;14:702–7.

8. Knockaert DC. Cardiac involvement in systemic inflammatory diseases. *Eur Heart J* 2007;28:1797–804.

9. Lancellotti P, Nkomo VT, Badano LP et al. Expert consensus for multi-modality imaging evaluation of cardiovascular complications of radiotherapy in adults: a report from the European Association of Cardiovascular Imaging and the American Society of Echocardiography. *J Am Soc Echocardiogr* 2013;26:1013–32.

10. Acquatella H. Echocardiography in Chagas heart disease. *Circulation* 2007;115:1124–31.

# Indications and appropriateness criteria for echocardiography

# 19

## 1 Contrast echocardiography[1-3]

### 1.1 Agitated saline or gelofusin

- Detecting a patent foramen ovale:
  - Stroke or TIA in a young subject (usually aged <50 years) or an older subject with suggestive clinical features
  - Diver
  - Unexplained severe hypoxia
- Improving incomplete tricuspid regurgitant signal for the estimation of pulmonary artery pressure
- Identification of persistent left sided SVC
- Identification of extracardiac shunt, e.g. pulmonary AV malformation

### 1.2 Transpulmonary contrast

- Poor LV endocardial definition:
  - Measurement of LV ejection fraction
  - Diagnosis of LV dysfunction
- Defining LV apical structures:
  - Thrombus
  - Apical hypertrophic cardiomyopathy
  - Noncompaction
- Indentifying pseudoaneuryms
- Stress echocardiography:
  - Poor endocardial definition
- Myocardial perfusion:
  - Early diagnosis of myocardial infarction
  - Improved detection of myocardial ischaemia
  - Detection of viability

## 2 Transoesophageal echocardiography[4, 5]

A non-exhaustive set of indications includes:

- Poor TTE image quality despite transpulmonary contrast as indicated
- Suspected endocarditis:
  - In most cases of replacement valve or implantable electrical device endocarditis
  - When the transthoracic study is non-diagnostic
- Cerebral infarction, transient ischaemic attack, peripheral embolism:
  - Patients aged <50 years with no identifiable non-cardiac source
  - Patients aged >50 years without evidence of cerebrovascular disease or other obvious cause in whom the findings of echocardiography will change management
- Initial evaluation of adult congenital disease
- Before cardioversion:
  - Previous cardioembolic event
  - Anticoagulation contraindicated or subtherapeutic
  - Atrial fibrillation of <48 hours' duration in the presence of structural heart disease
- Replacement heart valve:
  - To improve quantification of mitral regurgitation
  - Obstruction to determine the cause
  - Equivocal obstruction
  - Suspected endocarditis
  - Abnormal regurgitation suspected but transthoracic study normal or equivocal (breathless patient, hyperdynamic LV, haemolytic anaemia)
  - Recurrent thromboembolism despite adequate anticoagulation
- Native valve disease:
  - To determine feasibility and safety of balloon mitral valvotomy
  - To determine whether a regurgitant mitral valve is repairable
- Aorta:
  - To diagnose dissection, intramural haematoma or transection
  - To determine the size of the aorta
  - To measure the annulus diameter before a transcatheter procedure
- Perioperative:
  - To confirm preoperative diagnosis
  - To assess mitral valve repair
  - To confirm normal replacement valve function immediately after implantation
  - To confirm de-airing

- To detect myocardial ischaemia
- To assess the haemodynamically unstable patient on intensive care units
- Percutaneous procedures:
  - To assess before and to guide during transcatheter valve repairs and deployment of occlusion devices and crossing the atrial septum for RF ablation

## 3 Indications for stress echocardiography[5-10]

- Prediction of coronary disease in patients unsuitable for exercise ECG testing (e.g. resting ECG changes, unable to walk, exercise test likely to be inaccurate)
- Risk stratification in known coronary disease (e.g. after myocardial infarction)
- If clinically stable after acute chest pain with non-diagnostic ECG and normal or equivocal troponin
- After coronary angiography to assess functional significance of an equivocal lesion or after CT with equivocal calcium scores or angiography
- To determine the presence of viability in apparently infarcted myocardium
- LV dysfunction and coronary angiography not planned
- Before vascular surgery with coronary risk factors and poor or unknown functional capacity
- Symptoms after coronary revascularisation
- Low gradient low ejection fraction aortic stenosis
- Severe asymptomatic aortic stenosis, mitral stenosis or mitral regurgitation without resting thresholds for surgery
- Symptoms despite mild or moderate valve disease
- Preoperative assessment before high-risk non-cardiac surgery with poor or unknown functional capacity and clinical risk factors

## 4 Inappropriate indications for transthoracic echocardiography[11]

Assuming no change in clinical state, TTE is not usually indicated for the following conditions:

- **Arrhythmia** (with no clinical evidence of structural disease):
  - Infrequent atrial or ventricular ectopics
  - Sinus bradycardia
  - Light headedness or presyncope
- **LV function including cardiomyopathy:**
  - No symptoms or signs of cardiovascular disease including routine preoperative
  - Routine surveillance with known coronary disease

- Prior assessment with other techniques showing normal function
- Routine surveillance (<1 year) of heart failure with no change in clinical state
- Routine surveillance of an implanted device without change in clinical state
- Routine surveillance (>1 year) of known cardiomyopathy
- Routine surveillance in hypertension

- **Right heart:**
  - Suspected pulmonary embolism to establish the diagnosis
  - Surveillance of known PHT (<1 year)

- **Congenital:**
  - Routine surveillance (<2 years) after complete repair

- **General:**
  - Mild trauma with no ECG or troponin change
  - Routine surveillance of a small pericardial effusion with no change in clinical state
  - Known aortic dilatation if findings will not change management

- **Valve disease:**
  - Frequent surveillance in mild native valve disease. For recommended frequencies, see Table A3.4, page 222.
  - Transient fever with no bacteremia or a bacterium not associated with endocarditis
  - Routine surveillance of uncomplicated endocarditis

## References

1. Senior R, Becher H, Monaghan M et al. Contrast echocardiography: evidence-based recommendations by European Association of Echocardiography. *Eur J Echocardiogr* 2009;10:194–212.
2. Mulvagh SL, Rakowski H, Vannan MA et al. American Society of Echocardiography consensus statement on the clinical applications of ultrasonic contrast agents in echocardiography. *J Am Soc Echocardiogr* 2008;21:1179–201.
3. Stewart MJ. Contrast echocardiography. *Heart* 2003;89:342–8.
4. Flachskampf FA, Badano L, Daniel WG et al. Recommendations for transoesophageal echocardiography: update 2010. *Eur J Echocardiogr* 2010;11:557–76.
5. Sicari R, Nihoyannopoulos P, Evangelista A et al. Stress echocardiograpohy expert consensus statement. *Eur J Echocardiogr* 2008;9:415–37.
6. Becher H, Chambers J, Fox K et al. BSE procedure guidelines for the clinical application of stress echocardiography, recommendations for performance and interpretation of stress echocardiography: a report of the British Society of Echocardiography Policy Committee. *Heart* 2004;90 Suppl 6:vi23–vi30.

7.  Senior R, Monaghan M, Becher H, Mayet J, Nihoyannopoulos P, British Society of Echocardiography. Stress echocardiography for the diagnosis and risk stratification of patients with suspected or known coronary artery disease: a critical appraisal. *Heart* 2005;91(4):427–36.

8.  Pierard LA, Lancellotti. Stress testing in valve disease. *Heart* 2007;93:766–72.

9.  Pellikka PA, Nagueh SF, Elhendy AA et al. American Society of Echocardiography recommendations for performance, interpretation, and application of stress echocardiography. *J Am Soc Echocardiogr* 2007;20:1021–41.

10. Douglas PS, Khanderia B, Stainback RF et al. ACCF/ASE/ACEP/AHA/ASNC/SCAI/ SCCT/SCMR 2008. Appropriateness criteria for stress echocardiography. *Circulation* 2008;117:1478–97.

11. Douglas PS, Garcia MJ, Haines DE et al. ACCF/ASE/AHA/ASNC/HFSA/HRS SCAI/SCCM/ SCCT/SCMR 2011. Appropriateness criteria for echocardiography. *J Am Soc Echocardiogr* 2011;24:229–67.

# Appendices

## Appendix 1 Left ventricle

### A1.1 LV mass

- 3D and 2D methods of estimating mass are not widely used. An estimate can be made using linear dimensions at the base of the heart: using the approximation $0.83 \times [(LVDD + IVS + PW)^3 - LVDD^3]$
- A guide to grading is given in Table A1.1.

Table A1.1 Grading LV mass[1]

|  | Normal | Mild hypertrophy | Moderate hypertrophy | Severe hypertrophy |
|---|---|---|---|---|
| **Women** | | | | |
| LV mass (g) | 67–162 | 163–186 | 187–210 | ≥211 |
| LV mass/BSA (g/m²) | 43–95 | 96–108 | 109–121 | ≥122 |
| **Men** | | | | |
| LV mass (g) | 88–224 | 225–258 | 259–292 | ≥292 |
| LV mass/BSA (g/m²) | 49–115 | 116–131 | 132–148 | ≥149 |

### A1.2 Diastolic function

- LV diastolic function using flow propagation[2]
  - From a 4-chamber view, place the colour box over the mitral valve and the base of the LV. Place the cursor over the inflow signal. Reduce the velocity on the colour scale if necessary to ensure a clear aliasing signal in the red forward flow.
  - Use the calliper to draw a line about 4–5 cm long along the edge of the colour change and calculate the slope ($Vp$).
  - Divide this into the peak transmitral E wave velocity.
  - High filling pressures are suggested by a $Vp$/E ratio >1.8.

## A1.3 Cardiac resynchronisation optimisation

● Apart from measuring the ejection fraction (<35%) echocardiography is not useful to determine suitability for biventricular pacing[3] and currently the decision is made using the ECG.

● Echocardiography is not routinely used to optimise the pacemaker settings after implantation, but this may still be done in a patient with refractory symptoms.

● There is no consensus protocol, but this is a guide:

  ● Start with AV delay. Look at the size of the A wave and measure diastolic filling time and assess the grade of mitral regurgitation subjectively with:

    ● the shortest AV delay possible

    ● about 75 ms

    ● about 150 ms

    ● other intermediate delays as dictated by initial results.

  ● Choose the AV delay with the best developed A wave without shortening the A deceleration time and with the least mitral regurgitation.

  ● Then modify interventricular delay:

    ● both ventricles activated at the same time

    ● the right ventricle activated earlier than the left (e.g. 30 ms and 50 ms)

    ● the left ventricle activated earlier than the right (e.g. 30 ms and 50 ms).

  ● Choose the sequence with the highest subaortic velocity integral.

## A1.4 Deformation imaging

Strain is assessed by tissue Doppler or speckle-tracking. It has the promise of detection of early LV dysfunction for example after chemotherapy or in valve disease. Regional strain may detect coronary disease even relatively late after an episode of pain when no residual wall motion abnormality is obvious by eye. It is not yet established for routine clinical use since it is time-consuming and insufficient data are available. Data available are given in Tables A1.2 and A1.3.

Table A1.2 Normal ranges for strain imaging[4]

|  | 3D speckle tracking | 2D speckle tracking |
|---|---|---|
| Longitudinal % | −17.0 (5.5) | −19.9 (5.3) |
| Circumferential | −31.6 (8) | −27.8 (6.9) |

**Table A1.3** Reference values for 2D segmental longitudinal peak systole strain by speckle tracking (% and SD)[5]

| | | | | | |
|---|---|---|---|---|---|
| Basal septal | −13.7 (4.0) | Basal anterior | −20.1 (4.0) | Basal anteroseptal | −18.3 (3.5) |
| Mid septal | −18.7 (3.0) | Mid anterior | −18.8 (3.4) | Mid anteroseptal | −19.4 (3.2) |
| Apical septal | −22.3 (4.8) | Apical anterior | −19.4 (5.4) | Apical anteroseptal | −18.8 (5.9) |
| Apical lateral | −19.2 (5.4) | Apical inferior | −22.5 (4.5) | Apical posterior | −17.7 (6.0) |
| Mid lateral | −18.1 (3.5) | Mid inferior | −20.4 (3.5) | Mid posterior | −16.8 (5.0) |
| Basal lateral | −17.8 (5.0) | Basal inferior | −17.1 (3.9) | Basal posterior | −14.6 (7.4) |

# References

1. Lang RM, Bierig M, Devereux RB et al. Recommendations for chamber quantification. *Eur J Echocardiogr* 2006;7(2):79–108.
2. Takatsuji H, Mikami T, Urasawa K et al. A new approach for evaluation of left ventricular diastolic function: spatial and temporal analysis of left ventricular filling flow propagation by color M-mode Doppler echocardiography. *J Am Coll Cardiol* 1996;27(2):365–71.
3. Brignole M, Auricchio A, Baron-Esquivias G et al. 2013 ESC guidelines on cardiac pacing and cardiac resynchronisatin therapy. *Eur Heart J* 2013;34:2281–329.
4. Saito K, Okura H, Watanabe N et al. Comprehensive evaluation of left ventricular strain using speckle tracking echocardiography in normal adults: comparison of three-dimensional and two-dimensional approaches. *J Am Soc Echocardiogr* 2009;22(9):1025–30.
5. Marwick TH, Leano RL, Brown J et al. Myocardial strain measurement with 2-dimensional speckle-tracking echocardiography. *JACC Cardiovasc Imaging* 2009;2:80–4.

# Appendix 2 Critical care monitoring

## A2.1 Suitability for extracorporeal membrane oxygenation (ECMO)

Table A2.1 Suitability for ECMO*

| Reversible pathology avoiding ECMO |
| --- |
| Pericardial tamponade |
| Surgically correctible valve disease |
| **Absolute contraindications for venoarterial (VA) ECMO** |
| Severe aortic regurgitation |
| Unrepaired dissection |
| Widespread LV scarring |
| **Needs VA rather than veno-venous (VV) ECMO** |
| Severe LV impairment |
| Severe valve disease |
| **Contraindicates VV ECMO** |
| Severe PA hypertension (mean PA pressure >50 mmHg) |
| **Use peripheral rather than central lines** |
| Aortic atheroma |
| ASD, large PFO, atrial septal aneurysm |

*Veno-venous (VV) provides respiratory support for patients who are cardiologically stable.
Veno-arterial (VA) provides cardiac and respiratory support for patients who are cardiologically unstable

## A2.2 Monitoring ECMO

Table A2.2 Echocardiographic monitoring for ECMO[1]

| Confirm correct position of cannulae |
| --- |
| Access cannula near mouth of IVC |
| Return cannula in mid right atrium clear of interatrial septum and tricuspid valve |
| Incorrect positions include passing through a PFO or in the coronary sinus or RV |
| **General** |
| LV and RV function |
| MR |

| |
|---|
| Aortic valve opening |
| Pericardial fluid |
| **Complications** |
| Cannula displacement |
| Cannula thrombosis |
| Obstruction of veins or arteries |
| LV thrombus |
| Tamponade |
| Pulmonary embolism |
| Hypoxia from recirculation |

## A2.3 Weaning from ECMO

Table A2.3 Echocardiographic features supporting weaning from VA ECMO with flow reduction to <1.5 l/min[2, 3]

| |
|---|
| LVEF >20–25%[7, 8] and ideally >35%[6] |
| $VTI_{LVOT}$ ≥10 cm |
| Tissue Doppler peak systolic velocity ≥6 cm/s |
| Non-dilated LV |
| No cardiac tamponade |

## A2.4 Ventricular assist device

Table A2.4 Checklist for Impella temporary ventricular assist device*[4, 5]

| |
|---|
| **Before insertion** |
| LV size and function (diastolic volume <120 ml may limit effectiveness) |
| RV size and function |
| Grade of mitral and tricuspid regurgitation |
| *Contraindications* |
| Aortic pathology (dissection, abdominal or thoracic aortic aneurysm) |
| LV apical thrombus |
| Aortic stenosis or regurgitation |
| Small LV cavity, e.g. HCM |
| ASD |

(continued)

Table A2.4 Checklist for Impella temporary ventricular assist device*[4, 5] (*continued*)

| Contraindications |
| --- |
| Severe RV dysfunction (RV area change <20% may develop RV failure) |
| Severe pulmonary hypertension (systolic pressure >50 mmHg) |
| **At insertion** |
| Correct position (parasternal or apical long-axis view):<br>• Inlet area 40–45 mm below aortic valve<br>• Catheter angled towards the LV apex<br>• Catheter not curled up or obstructing the mitral valve or with the tip in the papillary muscle area |
| Colour Doppler mosaic flow pattern of the exit stream above the sinus of valsalva |
| Optimise left ventricular filling:<br>• Maximise E wave velocity and velocity integral<br>• Septal shift to right pump flow too low<br>• Septal shift to left pump flow too high |
| Exclude right to left atrial shunting |
| **Monitoring** |
| Verify position of catheter |
| Verify outflow mosaic pattern above the sinus of valsalva |
| Confirm permanently closed aortic and pulmonary valves |
| LV and RV systolic function:<br>• Echo-guided increase in pump speed for LV failure<br>• Echo-guided decrease in pump speed for RV failure |
| Ventricular unloading (transmitral E wave) |
| PA pressure |
| Grade of mitral regurgitation |
| Check for pericardial effusion |
| Exclude LV thrombus |

*Aspirates blood from the LV and ejects into the ascending aorta

# A2.5 Intra-aortic balloon pump

Table A2.5 Checklist for intra-aortic balloon pump

| **Contraindications** |
| --- |
| More than mild aortic regurgitation |
| Aortic pathology (severe atheroma, dissection, abdominal aneurysm) |

| Monitoring |
| --- |
| Correct position (tip at junction of arch and descending thoracic aorta) |
| No aortic regurgitation |
| Change in subaortic velocity integral with augmentation |
| Leakage (bubbles in aorta) |
| Exclude pericardial effusion |

# References

1. Platts DG, Sedgwick JF, Burstow DJ et al. The role of echocardiography in the management of patients supported by extracorporeal membrane oxygenation. *J Am Soc Echocardiogr* 2012;25:131–41.
2. Aissaoui N, Luyt CE, Leprince P et al. Predictors of successful extracorporeal membrane oxygenation (ECMO) weaning after assistance for refractory cardiogenic shock. *Intensive Care Med* 2011;37:1738–45.
3. Cavarocchi NC, Pitcher HT, Yang Q et al. Weaning of extracorporeal membrane oxygenation using continuous hemodynamic transesophageal echocardiography. *J Thorac Cardiovasc Surg* 2013;146:1474–9.
4. Mehrotra AK, Shah D, Sugeng L, Jolly N. Echocardiography for percutaneous heart pumps. *JACC Cardiovasc Imaging* 2009;2:1332–3
5. Catena E, Milazzo F, Merli M et al. Echocardiographic evaluation of patients receiving a new left ventricular assist device: the Impella recover 100. *Eur J Echocardiogr* 2004;5:430–7.

# Appendix 3 Valve disease

## A3.1 Mitral and tricuspid annulus diameters

Table A3.1 Mitral and tricuspid annulus diameters (mm) in systole[1]

|  |  |  | Indexed to BSA | |
|---|---|---|---|---|
|  | Male | Female | Male | Female |
| **Mitral** | | | | |
| Parasternal long-axis | 25–41 | 23–34 | 13–21 | 13–19 |
| 4-chambers | 25–38 | 23–33 | 13–19 | 13–19 |
| **Tricuspid** | | | | |
| 4-chambers | 23–34 | 20–34 | 12–17 | 11–19 |

## A3.2 Wilkins score

Table A3.2 Wilkins score[2]

| Morphology | Score* |
|---|---|
| **Mobility** | |
| Highly mobile, only tips restricted | 1 |
| Normal mobility of base and mid-leaflet | 2 |
| Valve moves forward in diastole mainly from the base | 3 |
| No or minimal movement | 4 |
| **Leaflet thickening** | |
| Near normal | 1 |
| Thickening mainly at tips | 2 |
| Thickening (5–8 mm) over the whole leaflet | 3 |
| Severe thickening (>8 mm) of whole leaflet | 4 |
| **Subvalvar thickening** | |
| Minimal just below leaflets | 1 |
| Over one third the chordate | 2 |
| Extending to the distal third of the chordate | 3 |
| Extensive thickening and shortening of the whole chord | 4 |

*A total score ≤8 suggests a successful result but the score has not been validated in a large population and does not assess some key points (see Table 8.3, page 79)

| Calcification | |
|---|---|
| A single area of echogenicity | 1 |
| Scattered areas at leaflet margin | 2 |
| Echogenicity extending to midportion of leaflets | 3 |
| Extensive echogenicity over whole leaflet | 4 |

## A3.3 Duke criteria for diagnosing infective endocarditis

Table A3.3 Duke clinical criteria for infective endocarditis[3]

| Major – Microbiological | Major – Echocardiographic | Minor |
|---|---|---|
| 1. Typical micro-organisms consistent with IE from two separate sets of blood cultures, e.g. oral streptococci, *Streptococcus bovis*, HACEK group, *Staphylococcus aureus* or community-acquired enterococci (in the absence of a primary focus) <br><br> OR <br><br> 2. Micro-organisms consistent with IE from persistently positive blood cultures: at least 2 positive blood cultures taken 12 h apart or all of 3 or a majority of 4 separate blood cultures (1 h between 1st and last samples) <br><br> OR <br><br> 3. Single positive blood culture for *Coxiella burnetti* or phase 1 IgG antibody titre 1:800 | 1. Vegetations <br><br> OR <br><br> 2. Abscess <br><br> OR <br><br> 3. Dehiscence of a prosthetic valve <br><br> OR <br><br> 4. Perforation of a valve <br><br> OR <br><br> 5. Fistula formation | 1. At risk heart condition, or IVDU <br><br> 2. Fever >38 °C <br><br> 3. Vascular phenomena: <br> • Emboli <br> • Septic pulmonary infarcts <br> • Intracranial haemorrhage <br> • Mycotic aneurysm <br><br> 4. Immunologic phenomena: <br> • Glomerulonephritis <br> • Rheumatoid factor <br> • Roth spots, etc. <br><br> 5. Microbiology other than major criteria |

Definite endocarditis is defined by 2 major or 1 major and 3 minor or 5 minor. Possible endocarditis is defined by 1 major or 3 minor.

# A3.4 Frequency of echocardiography in native valve disease

Table A3.4 Frequency of serial echocardiography for valve disease[4-6]

| Aortic valve disease | |
|---|---|
| Mild AS with little calcification | 2–3 years |
| Bicuspid with no AS or significant AR | 2–3 years |
| Moderate AS | 1 year |
| Moderate AS (>3.5 m/s) with heavy calcium | 6 months |
| Severe AS | 6 months |
| Mild AR | 3 year |
| Moderate AR | 2 year |
| Severe AR | Reassess in 6 months to determine rate of progression then 6-monthly if LVDD near 70 mm or SD 50 mm, otherwise 12-monthly |
| **Primary Mitral valve disease** | |
| Mild MR and normal MV | No follow-up usually needed |
| Mild MR and prolapse | 2–3 years |
| Moderate MR | 2 years |
| Severe MR close to cutpoints for surgery or no previous study | 6 months or less |
| Severe MR and normal LV | 1 year |
| **Right-sided valve disease** | |
| PS mild ($V_{max}$ <3 m/s) | 5 year |
| Moderate | 2 year |

# A3.5 Normal ranges for replacement heart valves: mean (standard deviation)

See Tables A3.5–A3.7. [4, 7, 8]

- Surprisingly little published data exist for normally functioning valves.
- The short and long form of the modified Bernoulli equation and the classical and modified versions of the continuity equation are used and account for some variation in results.
- Pressure half-time and the Hatle formula are not valid in normally functioning mitral prostheses and are omitted.

- Doppler results are broadly similar for valves sharing a similar design. For simplicity, results for one design in each category is given with a list of other valve designs for which data exist.
- Sizing conventions vary so it is possible that a given label size for a valve not on the list may not be equivalent to those that are. A change on serial studies is more revealing than a single measurement and the echocardiogram must be interprted in the clinical context.

**Table A3.5** Aortic position: biological

| | $V_{max}$ (m/s) | Peak $\Delta P$ (mmHg) | Mean $\Delta P$ (mmHg) | EOA (cm²) |
|---|---|---|---|---|
| **Stented porcine:** *Carpentier–Edwards standard as example (values similar for Carpentier–Edwards Supra-annular, Intact, Hancock I and II and Mosaic, Biocor, Epic)* | | | | |
| 19 mm | | 43.5 (12.7) | 25.6 (8.) | 0.9 (0.2) |
| 21 mm | 2.8 (0.5) | 27.2 (7.6) | 17.3 (6.2) | 1.5 (0.3) |
| 23 mm | 2.8 (0.7) | 28.9 (7.5) | 16.1 (6.2) | 1.7 (0.5) |
| 25 mm | 2.6 (0.6) | 24.0 (7.1) | 12.9 (4.6) | 1.9 (0.5) |
| 27 mm | 2.5 (0.5) | 22.1 (8.2) | 12.1 (5.5) | 2.3 (0.6) |
| 29 mm | 2.4 (0.4) | | 9.9 (2.9) | 2.8 (0.5) |
| **Stented bovine pericardial:** *Baxter Perimount as example (similar for Mitroflow, Edwards Pericardial, Labcor–Santiago, Mitroflow)* | | | | |
| 19 mm | 2.8 (0.1) | 32.5 (8.5) | 19.5 (5.5) | 1.3 (0.2) |
| 21 mm | 2.6 (0.4) | 24.9 (7.7) | 13.8 (4.0) | 1.3 (0.3) |
| 23 mm | 2.3 (0.5) | 19.9 (7.4) | 11.5 (3.9) | 1.6 (0.3) |
| 25 mm | 2.0 (0.3) | 16.5 (7.8) | 10.7 (3.8) | 1.6 (0.4) |
| 27 mm | | 12.8 (5.4) | 4.8 (2.2) | 2.0 (0.4) |
| **Homograft** | | | | |
| 22 mm | 1.7 (0.3) | | 5.8 (3.2) | 2.0 (0.6) |
| 26 mm | 1.4 (0.6) | | 6.8 (2.9) | 2.4 (0.7) |
| **Stentless** *Whole root as inclusion – St Jude Toronto (similar for Prima)* | | | | |
| 21 mm | | 22.6 (14.5) | 10.7 (7.2) | 1.3 (0.6) |
| 23 mm | | 16.2 (9.0) | 8.2 (4.7) | 1.6 (0.6) |
| 25 mm | | 12.7 (8.2) | 6.3 (4.1) | 1.8 (0.5) |
| 27 mm | | 10.1 (5.8) | 5.0 (2.9) | 2.0 (0.3) |
| 29 mm | | 7.7 (4.4) | 4.1 (2.4) | 2.4 (0.6) |

*(continued)*

Table A3.5 Aortic position: biological (*continued*)

|  | $V_{max}$ (m/s) | Peak $\Delta P$ (mmHg) | Mean $\Delta P$ (mmHg) | EOA (cm²) |
|---|---|---|---|---|
| *Cryolife–O'Brien (similar for Freestyle)* | | | | |
| 19 mm | | | 9.0 (2.0) | 1.5 (0.3) |
| 21 mm | | | 6.6 (2.9) | 1.7 (0.4) |
| 23 mm | | | 6.0 (2.3) | 2.3 (0.2) |
| 25 mm | | | 6.1 (2.6) | 2. 6 (0.2) |
| 27 mm | | | 4.0 (2.4) | 2.8 (0.3) |

$V_{max}$: peak velocity; $\Delta P$: pressure difference; EOA: effective orifice area

Table A3.6 Aortic position: mechanical

|  | $V_{max}$ (m/s) | Peak $\Delta P$ (mmHg) | Mean $\Delta P$ (mmHg) | EOA (cm²) |
|---|---|---|---|---|
| **Single tilting disc:** *Medtronic-Hall (similar values for Björk–Shiley monostrut and CC, Omnicarbon and Omniscience)* | | | | |
| 20 mm | 2.9 (0.4) | 34.4 (13.1) | 17.1 (5.3) | 1.2 (0.5) |
| 21 mm | 2.4 (0.4) | 26.9 (10.5) | 14.1 (5.9) | 1.1 (0.2) |
| 23 mm | 2.4 (0.6) | 26.9 (8.9) | 13.5 (4.8) | 1.4 (0.4) |
| 25 mm | 2.3 (0.5) | 17.1 (7.0) | 9.5 (4.3) | 1.5 (0.5) |
| 27 mm | 2.1 (0.5) | 18.9 (9.7) | 8.7 (5.6) | 1.9 (0.2) |
| **Bileaflet mechanical** | | | | |
| **Intra-annular:** *St Jude standard (similar for Carbomedics Standard, Edwards Mira, ATS, Sorin Bicarbon)* | | | | |
| 19 mm | 2.9 (0.5) | 35.2 (11.2) | 19.0 (6.3) | 1.0 (0.2) |
| 21 mm | 2.6 (0.5) | 28.3 (10.0) | 15.8 (5.7) | 1.3 (0.3) |
| 23 mm | 2.6 (0.4) | 25.3 (7.9) | 13.8 (5.3) | 1.6 (0.4) |
| 25 mm | 2.4 (0.5) | 22.6 (7.7) | 12.7 (5.1) | 1.9 (0.5) |
| 27 mm | 2.2 (0.4) | 19.9 (7.6) | 11.2 (4.8) | 2.4 (0.6) |
| 29 mm | 2.0 (0.1) | 17.7 (6.4) | 9.9 (2.9) | 2.8 (0.6) |
| **Intra-annular modified cuff or partially supra-annular:** *MCRI On-X (similar for St Jude Regent, St Jude HP, Carbmedics Reduced Cuff, Medtronic Advantage)* | | | | |
| 19 mm | | 21.3 (10.8) | 11.8 (3.4) | 1.5 (0.2) |
| 21 mm | | 16.4 (5.9) | 9.9 (3.6) | 1.7 (0.4) |

| | | | | |
|---|---|---|---|---|
| 23 mm | | 15.9 (6.4) | 8.6 (3.4) | 1.9 (0.6) |
| 25 mm | | 16.5 (10.2) | 6.9 (4.3) | 2.4 (0.6) |
| **Supra-annular:** *Carbomedics TopHat* | | | | |
| 21 mm | 2.6 (0.4) | 30.2 (10.9) | 14.9 (5.4) | 1.2 (0.3) |
| 23 mm | 2.4 (0.6) | 24.2 (7.6) | 12.5 (4.4) | 1.4 (0.4) |
| 25 mm | | | 9.5 (2.9) | 1.6 (0.3) |
| **Ball and cage:** *Starr–Edwards* | | | | |
| 23 mm | 3.4 (0.6) | 32.6 (12.8) | 22.0 (9.0) | 1.1 (0.2) |
| 24 mm | 3.6 (0.5) | 34.1 (10.3) | 22.1 (7.5) | 1.1 (0.3) |
| 26 mm | 3.0 (0.2) | 31.8 (9.0) | 19.7 (6.1) | |
| 27 mm | | 30.8 (6.3) | 18.5 (3.7) | |
| 29mm | | 29.3 (9.3) | 16.3 (5.5) | |

$V_{max}$: peak velocity; $\Delta P$: pressure difference; EOA: effective orifice area

**Table A3.7** Mitral position

| | $V_{max}$ (m/s) | Mean $\Delta P$ (mmHg) |
|---|---|---|
| **Stented porcine:** *Carpentier–Edwards (similar for Intact, Hancock)* | | |
| 27 mm | | 6.0 (2.0) |
| 29 mm | 1.5 (0.3) | 4.7 (2.0) |
| 31 mm | 1.5 (0.3) | 4.5 (2.0) |
| 33 mm | 1.4 (0.2) | 5.4 (4.0) |
| **Pericardial:** *Ionescu–Shiley (similar for Labcor–Santiago, Hancock pericardial, Carpentier–Edwards pericardial)* | | |
| 25 mm | 1.4 (0.2) | 4.9 (1.1) |
| 27 mm | 1.3 (0.2) | 3.2 (0.8) |
| 29 mm | 1.4 (0.2) | 3.2 (0.6) |
| 31 mm | 1.3 (0.1) | 2.7 (0.4) |
| **Single tilting disc:** *Björk–Shiley Monostrut (similar for Omnicarbon)* | | |
| 25 mm | 1.8 (0.3) | 5.6 (2.3) |
| 27 mm | 1.7 (0.4) | 4.5 (2.2) |
| 29 mm | 1.6 (0.3) | 4.3 (1.6) |
| 31 mm | 1.7 (0.3) | 4.9 (1.6) |

*(continued)*

Table A3.7 Mitral position (*continued*)

| | $V_{max}$ (m/s) | Mean $\Delta P$ (mmHg) |
|---|---|---|
| 33 mm | 1.3 (0.3) | |
| **Bileaflet:** *Carbomedics (similar for St Jude)* | | |
| 25 mm | 1.6 (0.2) | 4.3 (0.7) |
| 27 mm | 1.6 (0.3) | 3.7 (1.5) |
| 29 mm | 1.8 (0.3) | 3.7 (1.3) |
| 31 mm | 1.6 (0.4) | 3.3 (1.1) |
| 33 mm | 1.4 (0.3) | 3.4 (1.5) |
| **Caged-ball:** *Starr–Edwards* | | |
| 28 mm | 1.8 (0.2) | 7.0 (2.8) |
| 30 mm | 1.8 (0.2) | 7.0 (2.5) |
| 32 mm | 1.9 (0.4) | 5.1 (2.5) |

$V_{max}$: peak velocity; $\Delta P$: pressure difference

# References

1. Dwivedi G, Mahadevan G, Jimenez D, Frenneaux M, Steeds R. Reference values for mitral and tricuspid annular dimensions using two-dimensional echocardiography. *Echo Research and Practice* published September 1, 2014, doi:10.1530/ERP-14-0062.
2. Wilkins GT, Weyman AE, Abascal VM, Block PC, Palacios IF. Percutaneous balloon dilatation of the mitral valve: an analysis of echocardiographic variables related to outcome and the mechanism of dilatation. *Br Heart J* 1988;60:299–308.
3. Li JS, Sexton DJ, Mick N et al. Proposed modifications to the Duke criteria for the diagnosis of infective endocarditis. *Clin Infect Dis* 2000;30:633–8.
4. Zoghbi WA, Chambers JB, Dumesnil JG et al. American Society of Echocardiography recommendations for evaluation of prosthetic valves with two-dimensional and Doppler echocardiography. *J Am Soc Echo*cardiogr 2009;22:975–1014.
5. Lancellotti P, Tribouilloy C, Hagendorff A et al. European Association of Echocardiography recommendations for the assessment of valvular regurgitation. Part 2: mitral and tricuspid regurgitation (native valve disease). *Eur J Echocardiogr* 2010;11:307–32.
6. Vahanian A, Alfieri O, Andreotti F et al. Guidelines on the management of valvular heart disease (version 2012). *Eur Heart J* 2012;33:2451–96.
7. Rajani R, Mukherjee D, Chambers J. Doppler echocardiography in normally functioning replacement aortic valves: a review of 129 studies. *J Heart Valve Dis.* 2007;16(5):519–35.
8. Rosenhek R, Binder T, Maurer G, Baumgartner H. Normal values for Doppler echocardiographic assessment of heart valve prostheses. *J Am Soc Echocardiogr* 2003;16(11):1116–27.

# Appendix 4 Summary of formulae

## A4.1 Bernoulli equation

This equates potential and kinetic energy up- and downstream from a stenosis. The modified formula is used in two forms:

**Short modified Bernoulli equation:** $\Delta P = 4V_2^2$

**Long modified Bernoulli equation:** $\Delta P = 4(V_2^2 - V_1^2)$

where $\Delta P$ is transvalvar pressure difference, $V_1$ is subvalvar velocity, and $V_2$ is transvalvar velocity.

The short form can be used when subvalvar is much less than transvalvar velocity, e.g. mitral stenosis, moderate or severe aortic stenosis ($V_2$ >3.0 m/s), but NOT mild aortic stenosis or normally functioning replacement valves.

## A4.2 Continuity equation

This is used in two forms:

**The classical continuity equation:** $EOA = CSA \times VTI_{subaortic}/VTI_{ao}$

**The modified continuity equation:** $EOA = CSA \times V_1/V_2$

where EOA is effective orifice area, CSA is cross-sectional area of the left ventricular outflow tract, $VTI_{subaortic}$ and $VTI_{ao}$ are subaortic and transaortic systolic velocity integral. The modified form is only a reasonable approximation in significant aortic stenosis.

## A4.3 Pressure half-time

The pressure half-time orifice area formula is:

$$MOA = 220/T_{1/2}$$

where MOA is effective mitral orifice area (in $cm^2$) and $T_{1/2}$ is pressure half-time in ms. This formula should only be used in moderate or severe stenosis. It is not valid in normally functioning replacement valves.

## A4.4 Stroke volume and cardiac output

$$SV \text{ (in ml)} = CSA \times VTI_{subaortic}$$

where CSA is cross-sectional area of the left ventricular outflow tract (in $cm^2$), $VTI_{subaortic}$ is subaortic velocity integral (in cm).

$$\text{Cardiac output} = SV \times \text{heart rate}$$

## A4.5 Flow

**Flow (in ml/s) = CSA x VTI$_{subaortic}$ × 1000/SET**

where CSA is cross-sectional area of the left ventricular outflow tract (in cm$^2$), VTI$_{subaortic}$ is subaortic velocity integral (in cm), and SET is systolic ejection time (from opening to closing artifact of the aortic signal) (in ms).

## A4.6 Systemic vascular resistance

**Systemic vascular resistance = (mean arterial pressure × 80)/cardiac output**

where systemic vascular resistance is in dyne.sec/cm$^5$, mean arterial pressure is in mmHg and cardiac output is in l/min. Normal 800–1200 dyne.sec/cm$^5$.

## A4.7 Estimating normal or high systemic vascular resistance from mitral regurgitation and stroke distance[19]

A qualitative estimate of systemic vascular resistance is from: MR $V_{max}$/VTI$_{subaortic}$. A ratio >0.27 suggests high resistance and <0.2 suggests normal resistance.

## A4.8 Shunt calculation

Table A4.1 Chamber volume load and levels for shunt calculation

|  |  | Level for shunt calculation | |
| --- | --- | --- | --- |
|  | **Loaded chamber** | **Downstream** | **Upstream** |
| **ASD** | RV | Pulmonary artery | LV outflow |
| **VSD** | LV | Pulmonary artery | LV outflow |
| **PDA** | LV | LV outflow | Pulmonary valve |

- The stroke volume is calculated for the aortic valve as above (equation in A4.4) and then for the pulmonary valve using the diameter at the pulmonary annulus and the velocity integral calculated with the pulsed sample at the level of the annulus.
- If the annulus cannot be imaged reliably, the diameter of the pulmonary artery and the level for velocity recording should be taken downstream wherever possible.
- The shunt is then the ratio of the downstream to the upstream stroke volume (Table A4.1).

## References

1. Abbas AE, Fortuin FD, Patel B, Moreno CA, Schiller NB, Lester SJ. Noninvasive measurement of systemic vascular resistance using Doppler echocardiography. *J Am Soc Echocardiogr* 2004;17(8):834–8.

# Appendix 5 Figures

- Aortic dimensions by BSA (Figure A5.1)
- Aortic diameter at the sinotubular junction in tall subjects (Figure A5.2)
- Aortic diameter by age (Figure A5.3)
- Body surface nomogram (Figure A5.4)

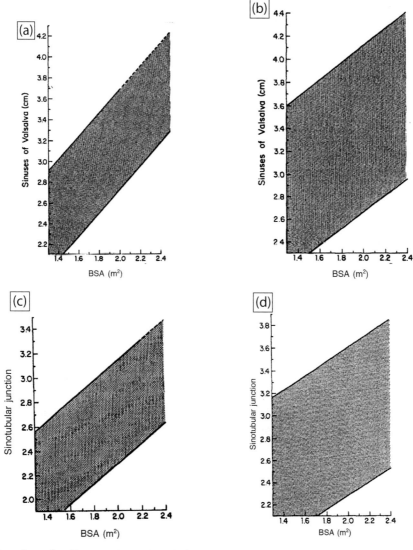

**Figure A5.1 Aortic dimensions by BSA.** (a) 95% range at the sinus for adults aged under 40 years (middle) and (b) adults aged 40 years and over (right). (c) 95% range at the sinotubular junction for adults aged under 40 and (d) adults aged 40 years and over (right). (Redrawn from Roman et al. 1989.[1])

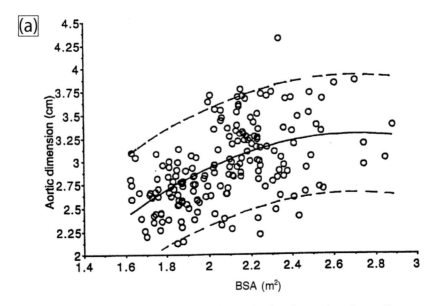

**Figure A5.2 Aortic diameter at the sinotubular junction in tall subjects.** Measurements were made using M-mode which is no longer recommended but may give a guide to the significance of 2D measurements. (Redrawn from Reed et al. 1993.[2])

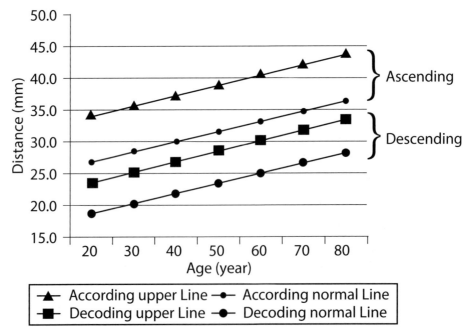

**Figure A5.3 Normal and upper limit diameter of ascending and descending thoracic aorta by age.** (Reproduced from Hannuksela et al. 2006.[3])

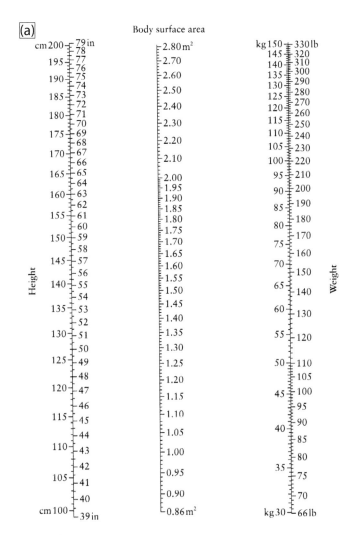

**Figure A5.4 Body surface nomogram.** Put a straight edge against the patient's height and weight and read off the body surface area on the middle column.

## References

1. Roman MJ, Devereux RB, Kramer-Fox R, O'Loughlin J. Two-dimensional echocardiographic aortic root dimensions in normal children and adults. *Am J Cardiol* 1989;64(8):507–12.
2. Reed CM, Rickey PA, Pullian DA, Somes GW. Aortic dimensions in tall men and women. *Am J Cardiol* 1993;71:608–10.
3. Hannuksela M, Lundqvist S, Carlberg B. Thoracic aorta: dilated or not? *Scan Cardiovasc J* 2006;40:175–8.

# Index